SECOND EDITION

INDICATIONS AND ALTERNATIVES IN X-RAY DIAGNOSIS

A Guide to the Effective Employment of Roentgenologic Studies in the Solution of Diagnostic Problems

MELVYN H. SCHREIBER, M.D.

Professor of Radiology
University of Texas Medical Branch
Galveston, Texas

CHARLES C THOMAS • PUBLISHER • SPRINGFIELD • ILLINOIS

Indications and Alternatives
in X-Ray Diagnosis

Second Edition

Indications and Alternatives in X-Ray Diagnosis

A Guide to the Effective Employment of Roentgenologic Studies in the Solution of Diagnostic Problems

By

MELVYN H. SCHREIBER, M.D.

Professor of Radiology
University of Texas Medical Branch
Galveston, Texas

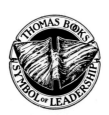

CHARLES C THOMAS · PUBLISHER
Springfield · Illinois · U.S.A.

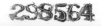

Published and Distributed Throughout the World by
CHARLES C THOMAS • PUBLISHER
Bannerstone House
301-327 East Lawrence Avenue, Springfield, Illinois, U.S.A.

© *1970 and 1974, by* CHARLES C THOMAS • PUBLISHER
ISBN 0-398-03027-8
Library of Congress Catalog Card Number: 73-16093

Printed in the United States of America
P-4

Library of Congress Cataloging in Publication Data

Schreiber, Melvyn H.
    Indications and alternatives in X-ray diagnosis.

    Bibliography: p.
    1. Diagnosis, Radioscopic.   I. Title.
[DNLM: 1. Radiography. WN200 S378i 1974]
RC78.S2226 1974   616.07'572   73-16093
ISBN 0-398-03027-8

To
Wes and Diane

PREFACE

THIS BOOK IS INTENDED for the medical student, general physician, and nonradiological specialist. It lists and discusses the kinds of x-ray examinations which are valuable in the study of different organ systems. Examples of the common abnormalities displayed by these different studies are presented, signs and symptoms of which constitute indications for the procedures. Such information should help the student and referring physician select the most appropriate radiologic examination to confirm or expose the suspected diagnosis, and where more than one study is available, the physician may present sensible alternatives to the patient.

There are many good general and special textbooks of radiology which describe and illustrate the abnormalities susceptible to radiologic demonstration. Some are listed in the Bibliography. This work is not an atlas or even a general text; it is a survey of radiologic diagnostic methods, arranged by organ systems, acquaintance with which will enable the physician to intelligently employ the appropriate test. In many cases the decision to perform a certain complex radiologic procedure will be made by a specialist consultant and not by the general physician. Often, the radiologist is in the best position to recommend and perform the indicated procedure. But the more the general physician and nonradiologic specialist know about the available radiologic alternatives, the better will they be able to direct the diagnostic approach to their patients' problems.

Other people who may find this volume interesting and valuable are the doctors' (and patients'!) helpers, sometimes, unfortunately, called paramedical personnel. They include the nurses, radiologic technologists, physical and occupational therapists, laboratory technicians, pulmonary therapists, medical record librarians, secretaries, administrators, clerks and typists, all of whom contribute in some way to patient care. While the physician must retain the ultimate authority and responsibility for choosing and employing diagnostic alternatives, informed helpers will materially improve the service the patient receives, the enthusiasm and dedication with which all of the members of the medical team perform, and the respect with which they view themselves and are viewed by others.

I am grateful to my colleagues for advice, criticism and encouragement, particularly to Drs. Robert N. Cooley, McClure Wilson, Luis Morettin and Charles Fagan. My secretary, Mrs. Tina Gourley, typed the manuscript many times and aided in numberless ways in its preparation. Lea & Febiger, publishers, granted permission to reproduce parts of Chapters 3 and 8 which previously appeared, in modified form, as articles in *The American Journal of The Medical Sciences.* The students of the University of Texas Medical Branch helped me to understand the need for such a book and provided the stimulation and excitement that make it fun to be a teacher.

MELVYN H. SCHREIBER

On the Strand
Galveston, Texas

PREFACE TO THE SECOND EDITION

THE ADDITION OF A NUMBER of carefully selected illustrations should substantially improve the usefulness of this introductory volume in roentgenology. An effort has been made to illustrate the appearances to be expected from most of the kinds of examinations discussed, and classical examples have usually been chosen. My object has been to familiarize the physician who orders x-ray examinations with what he can expect and to emphasize the alternatives available to him, to the roentgenologist and to the patient. It is as important to understand the limitations of these procedures as to appreciate the reasonable indications, and these have been emphasized at appropriate points in the text.

The Bibliography has been expanded and an Index has been added.

Milan Autengruber photographed the films and provided the prints used for the illustrations. Mrs. Tina Gourley provided secretarial assistance and support without which this Second Edition could not have been completed.

It is my hope that medical students, house officers, general and family physicians and nonradiological specialists will find this a useful guide in selecting x-ray studies, in seeking roentgenologic consultation and in organizing their thoughts about the diagnostic workup of their patients.

MELVYN H. SCHREIBER

Galveston, Texas

CONTENTS

Indications and Alternatives
in X-Ray Diagnosis

Chapter 1

THE SKELETAL SYSTEM

PLAIN FILMS

COMMON SENSE and a knowledge of anatomy will carry one a long way in the radiologic examination of bones. Plain films are ordinarily all that are required, and as long as one requests films focused on the area of interest and made at right angles to one another, little of importance will be missed. It is impressive how often a bony abnormality will be visible or at least be seen to good advantage in only one view (Figure 1). Considerable ingenuity must be exercised at times by the technician to obtain *two views at right angles to one another*. However, nothing less should be considered satisfactory.

The two views need not always be frontal and lateral views, however. If the patient is unable to move from the supine position and one is unable to place a film cassette behind the part of interest, oblique views of the part may prove quite satisfactory. In some situations, views with the x-ray beam angled toward the head or the feet may be of special value. An example is suspected fracture of the navicular of the wrist; ordinary frontal and lateral views may show no abnormality, while an angled view with the wrist abducted may show the fracture. In other circumstances the revealing views of a certain part may be frontal and oblique views, omitting the lateral, as in studies of the sacro-iliac joints. Some parts of the skeleton require a variety of films for careful display of suspected abnormalities. Examples are the lumbar spine (AP, lateral, oblique, and coned-down spot films) and the knee. AP and lateral views are routine, but the inter-condylar notch view ("tunnel" view) and the tangential view of the patella ("skyline" view) may be needed in certain instances.

For certain conditions *heavily exposed films* may be desirable or necessary. Osteoid osteomas and some other bone-producing or calcified tumors (Figures 2 and 3) may be so sclerotic that

3

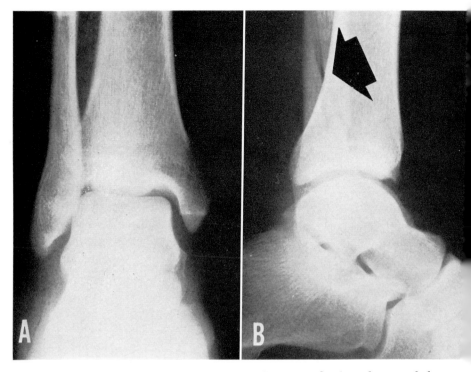

Figure 1. Fracture seen on one view only. In A, the frontal view of the ankle and distal leg, no abnormality is detected. On B, the lateral view made at right angles to the frontal view, the long oblique fracture of the fibula is easily seen (arrow). Two views at right angles are essential in searching for bony injuries.

overpenetrated films are required, and films made through plaster of paris casts may also require additional exposure. Under unusual circumstances *body section radiography* may be needed to see into the depths of a sclerotic lesion by blurring structures above and below the area of interest. When dealing with suspected facial fractures or in other circumstances where a three-dimensional image is important, *stereoscopic views* may be helpful.

Static films may be quite sufficient, depending upon the information sought. If the mobility of a joint is in question and particularly the bone and joint changes which accompany movement, then it may be desirable to obtain *films in flexion and extension,* particularly when dealing with the spine. Such films are

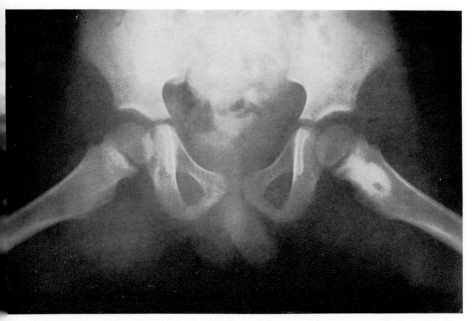

Figure 2. Osteoid osteoma. A classical sclerotic lesion with a radiolucent central nidus is seen in the proximal part of the left femur of this child. Overpenetrated views are sometimes necessary to demonstrate the nidus though such studies were not essential in this patient.

routine for inspection of the temporomandibular joint, where closed and open mouth films are regularly made. *Films in internal and external rotation* are used to study the shoulder and hip joints. In the patient with scoliosis it may be desirable to obtain films with the patient *supine* and *standing* as well as *films showing the effect of bending and tilting* to one side or another. Standing lateral films of patients suspected of having flat feet are necessary.

For the accurate determination of differences in lower extremity length (resulting from poliomyelitis, for example), special films are required. The extremity is immobilized alongside a measuring device. The central x-ray beam is sharply collimated, and three exposures are made on one film, the x-ray tube centered over the hip joint, the knee joint, and the ankle joint successively. The resulting film allows accurate measurement of the

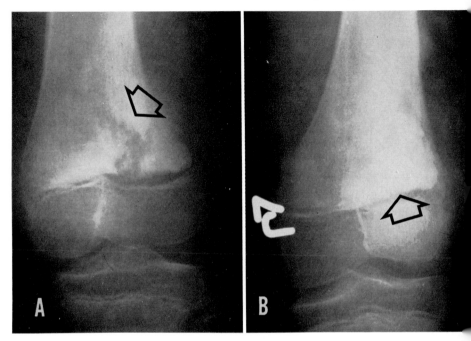

Figure 3 A and B. Osteosarcoma. In A the arrow points to a destructive lytic area in the distal femoral metaphysis. The arrow in B (a slightly oblique view) points to an area of increased bone production within the tumor producing a densely white sclerotic appearance.

femur and tibia for comparison with the other side and with the same side on serial studies.

Certain combinations of routine films are indicated in special circumstances. *The determination of bone age,* particularly in children, requires the exposure of certain kinds of films, depending upon what method is used. The simplest technique requires only the exposure of films of the hand and wrist or of the knee. Other methods require certain combinations of films, and in one method all of the secondary ossification centers on the left side of the skeleton are counted. As in most similar circumstances the method chosen is one with which the examiner is comfortable and experienced. All methods will produce usable information if carefully applied. A single determination of the skeletal age of a child is less likely to be accurate than an estimate resulting from serial determinations at several month intervals.

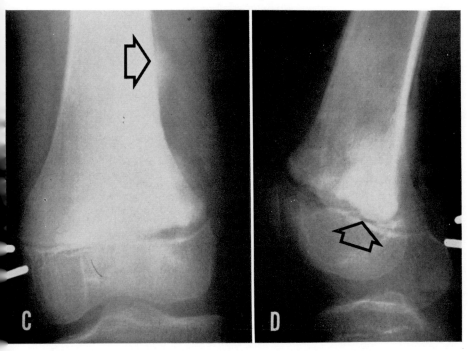

Figure 3 C and D. The arrow in C points to a typical Codman's triangle formed by elevation of the periosteum by the tumor and calcification and ossification within and beneath the elevated periosteum. The nearly lateral view (D) shows the mixed lytic and sclerotic nature of this typical osteogenic sarcoma occurring in the most common site, the distal femur.

Bone surveys are of value in other circumstances as well. Perhaps the "metastatic bone survey" is best known and most frequently ordered. It is a collection of films of the spine, proximal long bones, and skull and is used to search for evidence of metastatic deposits from a primary neoplasm elsewhere (Figure 4). It is probably ordered more often than it is needed to make decisions about therapy, particularly in patients known to have multiple myeloma. Other reasons for ordering skeletal surveys include dwarfism, osteogenesis imperfecta, suspicion of "battered child," multiple osteochondromas, and other generalized skeletal dysplasias.

With modern portable x-ray equipment, films of high quality can be made at the bedside or in the operating room, and Polaroid® films which can be viewed in seconds are also available.

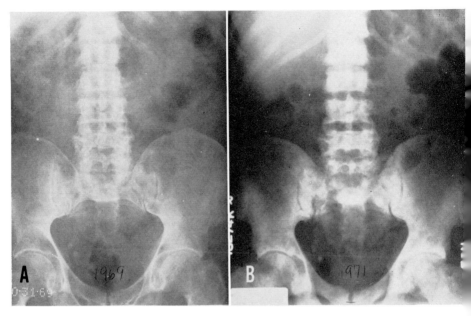

Figure 4. Metastatic prostatic carcinoma. (A) Frontal film of the abdomen exposed in 1969 shows no bony abnormality. (B) A similar film exposed two years later shows evidence of disseminated osteoblastic metastases from carcinoma of the prostate. The first and second lumbar vertebrae are particularly affected and are densely white, and one can see similar areas of increased density in the sacrum, in the innominate bones and in the proximal femurs.

Portable films should never be considered a substitute for films made in the Radiology Department if the latter can be obtained.

FLUOROSCOPY AND CINEFLUOROGRAPHY

Many tragic accidents occurred in the early days of the use of roentgen rays because of excessive exposure to the operator's hands during the reduction of fractures. The development of image amplification has substantially reduced the amount of x-ray energy necessary to produce a visible fluoroscopic image and has reduced the danger, but fluoroscopy for the reduction of fractures has been abandoned in most centers and is to be condemned as still hazardous. Fracture reduction can be monitored quite satisfactorily with conventional, portable, or Polaroid films, exposing the operator to little or no radiation hazard.

Image-amplified fluoroscopy may at times be used in monitoring closely the placement of a needle within the bone marrow for aspiration biopsy or for the injection of contrast material for intraosseous venography. Such needles may be safely placed in numerous locations, such as the greater trochanter of the femur, spinous processes of vertebrae, and ribs, and placement rarely requires film monitoring of any sort. Occasionally, fluoroscopic direction may be desirable, but even under these circumstances it should be used sparingly.

Fluoroscopy and cinefluorography are of questionable value for the study and display of joint motion and mobility. The cervical spine has been examined extensively in this way. While one can gain considerable knowledge of the mobility of the various cervical segments by cinefluorography in patients with degenerative joint disease, old injuries, or following operations for fusion, it is doubtful that more is learned than conventional flexion and extension films display. On rare occasions short x-ray movie strips of other joints in motion may provide valuable information but are seldom used.

ARTHROGRAPHY

Under aseptic conditions, contrast material may be deposited within joints, and after allowing time for mixing and diffusion, films may be exposed in various projections. Numerous films are usually made, with the part in flexion and extension, from various angles, and under various stresses. Most often, arthrography is performed for the detection of cartilaginous tears and imperfections, and the knee joint is more often examined than any other (Figure 5). Arthrography may also be used to determine the integrity of the joint space following fracture and to examine abnormalities of the synovial membrane.

ANGIOGRAPHY

Arteriography may be of considerable value in the study of abnormalities of the skeletal system. Certain fractures are commonly associated with vascular injuries, and early arteriography following the injury may indicate the need for operative vascular repair. Gunshot wounds and other injuries of the soft parts of the extremities which do not produce fracture may nonetheless

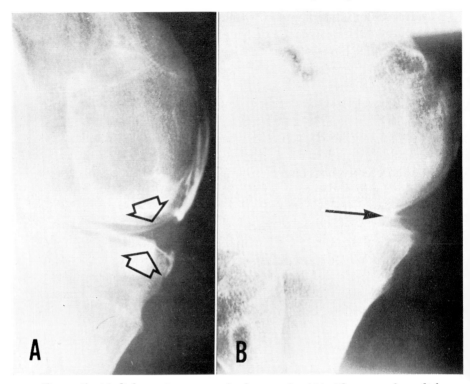

Figure 5. Medial meniscus tear (arthrogram). (A) The normal medial meniscus, to which the arrows point, appears as a triangular radiolucent area between the medial tibial plateau and the medial femoral condyle. (B) A horizontal tear of the medial meniscus is seen on an arthrogram as an area into which the contrast material dissects (arrow), producing a disruption of the usually perfectly smoooth triangular radiolucency of the cartilage which makes up the medial meniscus.

produce vascular injury requiring arteriography for demonstration and for the planning of appropriate therapy. Congenital anomalies such as arteriovenous malformations of bone and adjacent soft tissues lend themselves particularly well to arteriographic demonstration.

Tumors of bone are seldom studied arteriographically but may at times require such a procedure. One particularly difficult distinction is that between acute osteomyelitis and predominantly lytic osteosarcoma. Under these circumstances an arteriogram showing tumor vessels and tumor stain may be of decisive value. Arteriography is also useful in the study of soft tissue masses connected with or adjacent to bones, such as soft tissue sarcomas or benign tumors such as lipomas and fibromas of the extremities. Arteriography shows characteristic changes in many of these lesions, particularly the soft tissue sarcomas, and can lead to a precise diagnosis (Figure 6). Arteriography can also

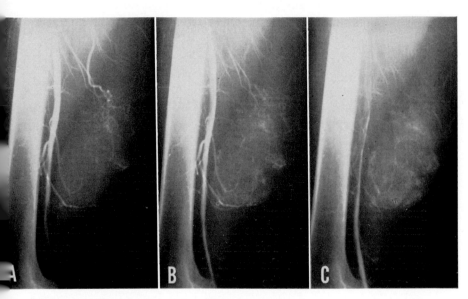

Figure 6. Fibrosarcoma of the thigh (arteriogram). Arteriography in this large mass on the posterior aspect of the midportion of the thigh shows, in A, tortuous vessels of increased caliber and irregular contour supplying the lesion. A slightly later film in this serial study (B) shows early puddling of the contrast agent in irregular vascular spaces. A later film in the sequence (C) shows that most of the contrast material has left the arteries and is now collected in sizable lakes within this typically vascular malignant mesodermal neoplasm.

define the limits of the lesion or indicate the likeliest spot for a diagnostic biopsy (a vascular portion of the leading edge of the tumor).

Venography, by the intravenous or intraosseous route, may provide information regarding venous obstruction following injuries or after an episode of thrombophlebitis. It may demonstrate vascular tears or show the presence of varicosities, particularly of the lower extremity. It is rarely employed for other reasons and has little value in the study of tumors or infections of bone.

Lymphangiography is thought by some to be useful in the investigation of chronic edema of the extremities. It may show lymphatic obstruction and ectasia. The therapeutic implications of a positive lymphangiogram in chronic leg edema are few unless a major plastic reconstructive operation is anticipated.

MYELOGRAPHY

Oily opaque iodinated contrast material is ordinarily employed, but air myelography may also be performed. The contrast substance is usually introduced by lumbar puncture into the subarachnoid space, but it may also be administered through cisternal puncture.

Abnormalities of and related to the skeletal system susceptible to display by myelography include herniated nucleus pulposus (Figure 7) and a variety of tumors and anomalies. Bony protrusions such as osteophytes may deform the oil column, and tumors of bone may produce deformities and obstruction. More commonly, defects and deformities resulting from tumors are the result of metastases to the vertebral canal and its contents. Lesions which arise from the central or peripheral nervous system, including tumors of the spinal cord, of its coverings, and of nerve roots and their sleeves as they exit through the intervertebral foramina, may also produce myelographic deformities and obstructions. Finally, myelography may display congenital vascular abnormalities such as arteriovenous malformations and may show defects secondary to infection of the meninges, particularly arachnoiditis.

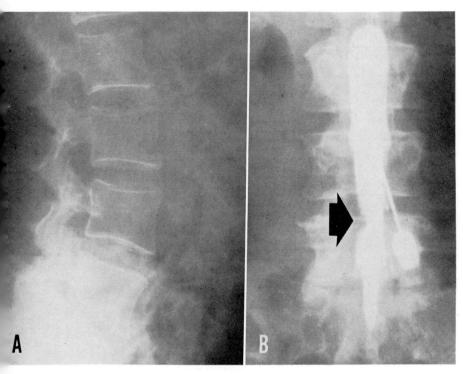

Figure 7. Herniated lumbar intervertebral disc (myelogram). The lateral film of the lumbar spine (A) shows no abnormality (and need not show even joint space narrowing in the presence of a herniated nucleus pulposus). The lumbar myelogram (B) shows a notch-like defect (arrow) produced by the extradural impression of the herniated disc material upon the opacified lumbar subarachnoid space. Observe that the defect is located almost exactly at the intervertebral space between the fourth and fifth lumbar vertebrae.

Chapter 2

THE SKULL, FACIAL BONES, PARANASAL SINUSES, MASTOIDS AND TEMPORAL BONES, AND THE CENTRAL NERVOUS SYSTEM

THE SKULL

THE ROUTINE OR ORDINARY views of the skull usually consist of the following: posteroanterior view, angled anteroposterior (Towne's) view, and right and left lateral views. At times the basal view is considered part of the routine study, and some radiologists prefer stereo lateral views. The routine views will be found to be quite satisfactory for the large majority of suspected abnormalities of the skull. Special views of the base, the petrous ridge, the optic foramina, the temporomandibular joints, and the sella turcica should be specifically requested when indicated. At times *stereoscopic views* of the skull may be valuable in localizing intracranial abnormalities, particularly calcifications but also foreign bodies, and *body section radiography* may at times be needed to verify the presence or define the extent of an abnormality. Abnormalities in and about the sella turcica may require body section radiography for elucidation, particularly asymmetrical erosion of the floor or of the dorsum sellae and calcifications superimposed upon the sella and seen in the routine lateral projections only. *Oblique and tangential views* may be useful for examining bony abnormalities, but *coned-down views* will not often be necessary (they are elegant when properly done and demonstrate the technician's marksmanship, but it is doubtful if one can see more on a coned-down view of a part of the skull than on a full-sized view in the same projection). One possible exception is coned-down basal views of the external auditory canal and middle ear when searching for the ossicles of the middle ear.

The kinds of abnormalities of the skull susceptible to diag-

14

nosis by x-ray examination may be conveniently divided into the following four categories. Signs and symptoms of the abnormalities described constitute indications for films of the skull.

Changes in Size

The size of the skull may be increased in acromegaly (the sella turcica, paranasal sinuses, and mandible may also be enlarged), Paget's disease, and hydrocephalus in childhood resulting from chronic increased intracranial pressure. The size of the skull may be decreased in cerebral dysgenesis or hypoplasia (congenital microcephaly), since the growth of the skull parallels and for the most part depends upon continued increase in the size of the brain. The skull may be decreased in size in premature closure of the cranial sutures, but unless all of the sutures have fused prematurely, the more likely result is an abnormality of shape than genuine diminution in volume.

Changes in Shape

The skull may be distorted by trauma of several sorts. Depressed skull fractures (Figure 8) and gross avulsion injuries obviously alter the shape of the skull. Positional "trauma" resulting from failure of a child to move his head, thereby lying always in the same position (because of brain damage, for example), may result in flattening of the skull. Distortion, particularly flattening, may also be due to softening of the skull, resulting from osteomalacia (rickets, for example). The skull cannot grow perpendicular to cranial sutures which are prematurely fused, and premature cranial synostosis results in distortion on that basis. If the coronal suture closes prematurely, the skull cannot grow in length from front to back, and a high, wide, short skull results. If the sagittal suture fuses early, the skull cannot grow in width from side to side, and an elongated narrow skull results. Since the shape of the skull depends in large measure upon the shape of the brain, congenital hemiatrophy of the brain can produce distortion of the skull. The distortion is internal as well as external, producing enlargement of the temporal bone, overgrowth of sinuses, and thickening of the diploë on the affected side.

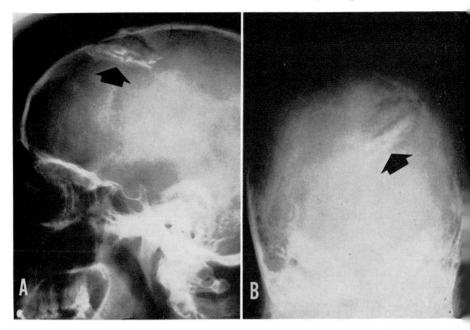

Figure 8. Depressed skull fracture. In the lateral view (A) and the Towne's view (B), the arrow points to an area of *increased* density representing the overlapping bone edges resulting from depression of a fragment of calvarium. Ordinary skull fractures appear as linear radiolucent lines, but depressed skull fractures show an area of decreased density where the bone has been avulsed and increased density where superimposition of the fragments and normal calvarium occurs.

Expanding lesions of the skull, its coverings, and its contents may also distort the shape of the skull. These mostly consist of tumors, benign and malignant, of the skull, scalp, paranasal sinuses, facial bones, and rarely, the brain. Other uncommon abnormalities such as mucoceles of the sinuses and fibrous dysplasia may produce abnormalities of the shape of the skull.

Changes in Mineralization

Generalized decrease in mineralization of the skull is found in osteoporosis (for example, postmenopausal, steroid administration) and osteomalacia (for example, rickets, malabsorption, chronic renal failure). Localized diminution in mineralization of the skull may be caused by many more conditions than the generalized type. One of the most common causes of localized loss of skull substance, particularly in older people, is metastatic carcinoma. Multiple myeloma also produces multiple localized lytic lesions of the skull (Figure 9). When sharply demarcated,

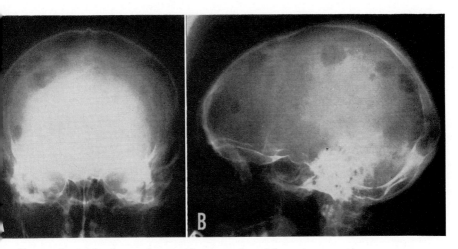

Figure 9. Multiple myeloma. The frontal and lateral views show numerous large and small clearly defined "punched-out" bony defects in the skull characteristic of multiple myeloma. Metastatic carcinoma may occasionally produce such a finding, and in a child or younger person, reticuloendotheliosis should be considered.

large and small, well-defined skull defects are found in young people, one of the reticuloendothelioses should be considered. Osteomyelitis of the skull produces localized loss of substance, though if it is chronic, it may also be accompanied by some sclerosis. Primary tumors of the skull such as osteogenic sarcoma are locally destructive, and tumors of the brain and meninges (particularly the latter) may cause erosion of the skull. Vascular malformations may produce serpiginous defects in the inner table and diploë of the skull, and prominent but normal foramina for emissary veins cause diminished localized mineralization. Skull defects produced by vascular lakes in the diploë and by erosion from arachnoidal granulations are also common and at times cause considerable diagnostic difficulty.

The overall mineralization of the skull may be increased in

osteopetrosis, fluoride intoxication, and chronic anemia. Localized increase in opacity of the skull may be the result of chronic osteomyelitis, Paget's disease, metastatic carcinoma (more often produces lytic lesions), tumors of the skull (osteomas), tumors of the meninges, fibrous dysplasia, and depressed skull fractures (resulting from the overlapping edges of the depressed fragment and the adjacent normal skull).

Changes in Character of Bony Architecture

The most common cause of disruption of the normal bony architecture of the skull is trauma. The diagnosis of skull fracture usually depends upon the demonstration of a linear or stellate radiolucency at or near the point of impact. Fractures at a distance from the point of impact (*contrecoup* injuries) are also common, and all fractures of the base of the skull are of this type. When sizable, fractures present no diagnostic problem. Fractures of the base are unusually difficult to diagnose, however. A lateral film of the skull with the x-ray beam projected horizontally is recommended in all cases of suspected basal skull fracture in order to determine the presence of a fluid level in the sphenoid sinus, a strong clue to the presence of such an injury. If the meninges are caught between the edges of a skull fracture in a young child, a leptomeningeal cyst may result weeks or months later because of pulsation of the underlying brain and eventual erosion and enlargement of the margins of the fracture line.

A few small wormian bones may normally be found in the lambdoidal suture. When they are markedly increased in number, and particularly when large portions of the skull consist of small patches of ossification rather than the formation of sheetlike cranial bones, the following diagnostic possibilities should come to mind: cretinism, cleidocranial dysostosis, osteogenesis imperfecta, and arrested hydrocephalus.

Diffuse thickening of the vault of the skull, leaving the inner table relatively intact, may be found in chronic anemias and in acromegaly. The hemolytic anemias, if severe, may also produce a "hair on end" appearance in the skull, as may the localized lesion of hemangioma.

Increased convolutional markings may be due to chronically increased intracranial pressure and increased intracranial pressure in childhood which has subsequently been relieved, spontaneously or otherwise. Lacunar skull (craniolacunia) may also produce convoluted impressions on the inner table. This abnormality is commonly associated with meningomyelocele. The range of normal in the appearance of the convolutional markings of the skull is considerable, and care should be taken not to mistake normal variation for an abnormality.

Periosteal proliferation in the skull may be found in infection, following injury (particularly cephalhematoma in newborns), and in healing rickets. Osteogenic sarcoma may occasionally elevate the periosteum, but metastases and multiple myeloma do not.

THE FACIAL BONES

Since one is ordinarily interested in displaying a specific abnormality when ordering x-ray films of the face, specific views should be requested, or the abnormality sought should be conveyed to the radiologist so that he may order the appropriate views. The Water's view is by far the most generally useful. Films of the nasal bones include posteroanterior, lateral, and superior-inferior views, often utilizing dental films. Tangential views may also be obtained. Films of the mandible include anteroposterior and individual oblique views, though occasionally basal and Towne's views may be helpful. Posteroanterior and lateral views of the orbits are usual, and special views of the optic foramina may be made when indicated (symptoms suggesting abnormalities which produce enlargement, such as optic glioma, or constriction, such as Paget's disease, fibrous dysplasia, and meningioma). Special methods also exist for the radiographic localization of opaque foreign bodies within the orbit. The usual views of the zygomatic arches are the angled posteroanterior view (Water's view) and the underexposed basal view.

The only three abnormalities encountered with any frequency on films of the face are fractures (linear, stellate, diastatic), infections and tumors. Fibrous dysplasia and Paget's disease may rarely produce sclerotic deformities of the facial bones. Abnormalities of the teeth and the adjacent bone in which they are embedded may also be displayed on appropriate films of the face, but these are more often handled by dentist and oral surgeon than by the radiologist. Stones in the salivary glands or ducts may be shown on routine films, and sialography with opaque contrast substance may be indicated when visualization of the parenchyma or ducts is desirable (masses, infections, and so forth).

THE PARANASAL SINUSES

The routine views of the paranasal sinuses are the Caldwell view, the Water's view (an angled posteroanterior projection), the lateral view, and the basal view. The only special views of the paranasal sinuses which are likely to be valuable are those produced by body section radiography when blurring of the structures in front of and behind a suspected abnormality is desired in order to focus more sharply on the area of interest. Suspicion of destruction of the bony walls of a sinus by spread of a malignant neoplasm is the usual indication. The optic foramen view is useful for study of the ethmoid sinuses.

The paranasal sinuses are often increased in size in acromegaly. Mucoceles may enlarge the sinus cavities but are almost limited to the frontal sinuses. The sinuses may be diminished in size because of underdevelopment, and complete absence (aplasia) of the frontal sinuses is a common finding.

Aeration of the paranasal sinuses may be diminished by many abnormalities. The mucous membrane lining the sinus cavities may be thickened by infection or by allergic edema (Figure 10). Transudation of fluid into the sinuses may accompany head colds, the common cold, or other infections. Pyogenic infections may result in the presence of pus within the sinuses, and if the films are made with a horizontal x-ray beam, an air-fluid level may be detected and aid in the diagnosis. Opacity of the sinuses following trauma is commonly due to bleeding into them and may or may not be associated with a fracture of the sinus wall. That is particularly true of the maxillary sinuses following trauma to the face. Spinal fluid may leak into the sphenoid sinus following

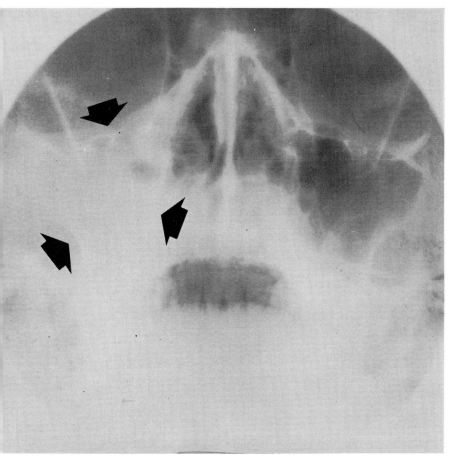

Figure 10. Right maxillary sinusitis. The Water's view of the face shows a normal maxillary sinus on the left. On the right the maxillary sinus is almost completely opaque (arrows), but its bony walls are intact. The lumen is filled with thickened mucous membrane and purulent material.

basal skull fracture, and a lateral film with a horizontal beam is important when that is suspected.

The sinuses commonly contain rounded soft tissue nodules which represent benign retention cysts. Polyps also occur in the sinuses but are usually associated with thickened mucous membrane and are usually on an allergic basis. Carcinoma of the sinuses also produces a clouding of the sinus cavity, and a clue to the diagnosis is the occurrence of bony destruction of one or more sinus walls. Osteomas of the frontal or ethmoid sinus are a common and ordinarily inconsequential occurrence.

Interruption or destruction of the walls of the paranasal sinuses are an important diagnostic clue. Most often, fractures, malignant neoplasms, or osteomyelitis will be responsible.

When plain films of the sinuses are inconclusive regarding the presence of a mass, opaque material may be introduced and the lesion sought for as a filling defect.

MASTOIDS AND TEMPORAL BONES

With regard to the temporal bone it is difficult to say where routine views leave off and special views begin, since each of the positions is relatively complex and requires special care in positioning. The views ordinarily employed include Towne's view, Law's view, Stenver's view, Mayer's view and Schüller's view. Each of these exposes the temporal bone and mastoid area to inspection from a slightly different angle.

Films of the temporal bones and mastoids are ordinarily made in the search for evidence of infection and occasionally for tumor. Increased density of the mastoid area suggests chronic mastoiditis as does the inadequate development of air cells on one side relative to the other. A localized area of diminished density, particularly if it is discrete and surrounded by a sclerotic zone, suggests cholesteatoma.

If the mastoids are normally formed and comparable on the two sides, a diminution in the extent of aeration and destruction of bony walls suggests that the mastoid air cells contain thickened mucous membrane (evidence of infection), pus, blood (history of trauma?), or tumor.

Because it provides passage for the eighth nerve, the internal auditory meatus and canal are of special interest. A small range of normal in size and shape exists, and precise symmetry is not always seen. Widening of the internal auditory canal with erosion of the adjacent bony margins suggests the presence of an eighth nerve tumor or rarely a glomus jugulare tumor.

Body section radiography is especially valuable in the study of abnormalities of the temporal bone. Sophisticated equipment capable of making "cuts" less than one millimeter thick may permit the exposure of films which display with exquisite clarity and detail the anatomy of the middle and inner ear.

THE CENTRAL NERVOUS SYSTEM

The Brain

Of the numerous methods of study of the brain, the simplest is plain films of the skull. Such films may demonstrate abnormal calcifications within the brain, bony changes secondary to diseases or abnormalities of the brain or meninges (meningioma for example), and widened sutures, enlargement of the sella, and increased convolutional markings indicating increased intracranial pressure.

Of the special techniques for radiographic examination of the brain, *pneumoencephalography* is indicated (a) for study of lesions of the brain stem, basal ganglia, and basilar cisterns (Figure 11); (b) for lesions of the posterior fossa; and (c) for atrophic lesions of the cerebrum (porencephalic cysts, for example). This examination utilizes air, ordinarily injected into the lumbar subarachnoid space, as contrast material. The central nervous system chambers are outlined by variously positioning the patient. *Ventriculography* (the direct injection of contrast material into the ventricular system) with air is indicated for study of the same conditions as indicated above under pneumoencephalography when increased intracranial pressure is present. Ventriculography may also be performed with opaque material. Opaque oil is sometimes used in very small amounts for better definition of lesions of the third and fourth ventricles and the aqueduct of Sylvius, particularly when air has produced an inadequate study. Aqueous iodinated contrast materials (particularly Conray®-60) have also been employed for opacification of the ventricles, but the procedure is still experimental.

Carotid arteriography is utilized for the study of (a) mass lesions of the cerebrum and its meninges (Figure 12) and (b) for lesions which are primarily vascular in nature, such as aneurysms, arteriovenous malformations, vascular occlusions, arterio-

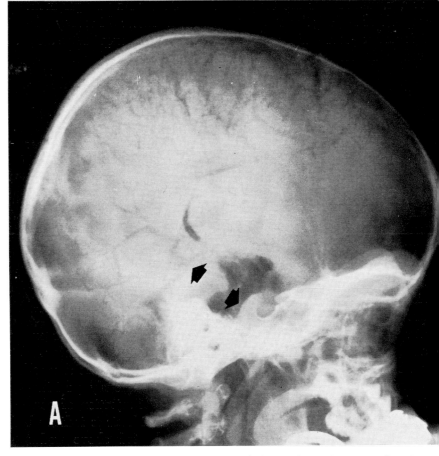

Figure 11. Pontine tumor (pneumoencephalogram). In A, a normal patient included for comparison, one sees a normal distance between the posterior part of the dorsum sellae and the upper floor of the fourth ventricle where it joins the aqueduct of Sylvius.

sclerosis and hematomas (Figure 13). A variety of techniques is available for the performance of carotid arteriography. The usual method of study is by direct percutaneous common carotid artery puncture and injection of contrast material. The carotid arteries may also be catheterized by way of the arteries of either arm or either leg.

Vertebral arteriography is employed for the study of sus-

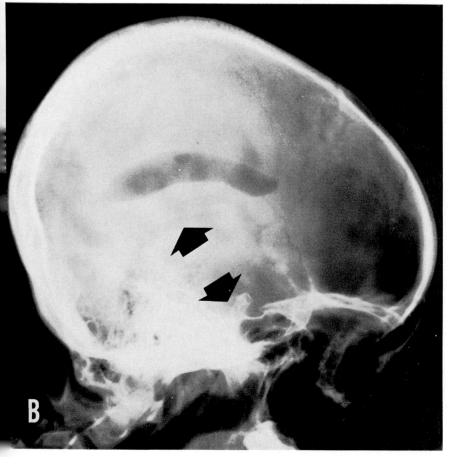

Figure 11 B. In B this distance is greatly increased by the presence of a neoplasm in the pons, and the faintly seen fourth ventricle and aqueduct are bowed posteriorly and superiorly by enlargement of the pons.

pected vascular lesions of the posterior fossa (Figure 14). Several techniques are available for this kind of examination. Direct percutaneous puncture of the vertebral arteries is hazardous and has been abandoned in many centers. Retrograde countercurrent brachial arteriography may be effective in opacifying the vertebral arteries and the posterior fossa, and the vertebral arteries may be catheterized from below by sophisticated techniques.

For the study of vascular lesions involving the origins of the

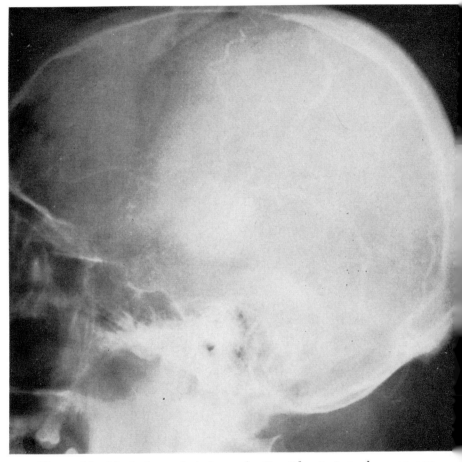

Figure 12. Meningioma (arteriogram). Carotid arteriography was performed and serial films were exposed. This is a late film from the series after the intracranial arteries have emptied (the capillary phase). In the temporo-parietal region one sees a rounded tumor "stain" characteristic of meningioma and produced by the suffusion of contrast material through the vascular spaces of this neoplasm. Such a homogeneous tumor stain is almost diagnostic of meningioma.

great vessels to the head and neck, *"four-vessel arteriography"* is indicated. This is performed by introducing a catheter into the ascending aorta, ordinarily by way of percutaneous puncture of the femoral artery, and the injection of a large volume of contrast material (about 60 cc) followed by serial filming in the right

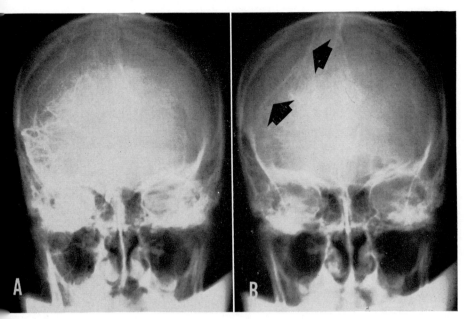

Figure 13. Subdural hematoma (carotid arteriogram). The arterial phase is shown in A. On this film one sees displacement of the anterior cerebral artery toward the left across the midline and failure of the intracranial branches of the middle cerebral artery to reach the inner table of the skull. In B, the venous phase, the midline displacement is again displayed. The arrows point to the clearly defined edge of the lenticular subdural hematoma, made visible by inward displacement of venous structures on the surface of the brain.

posterior oblique projection. This method opacifies both common carotid arteries and the origins of both internal carotid and external carotid arteries as well as both vertebral arteries throughout their course.

Unilateral internal jugular *venography* is rarely performed but may be indicated in patients with acoustic neuroma. Demonstration of the expected connection between the sigmoid and lateral venous sinuses on one side with those on the other side allows the surgeon to sacrifice those on the side of the tumor if necessary during resection of the tumor. Glomus jugulare tumors may protrude into and appear as filling defects within the internal jugular vein.

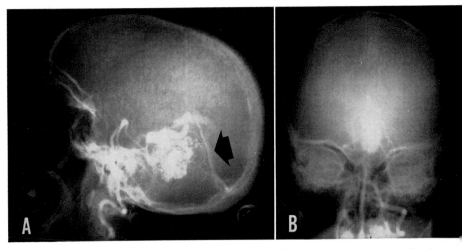

Figure 14. Posterior fossa arteriovenous malformation (arteriogram). A vertebral arteriogram has been performed and the lateral view is seen in A. A tangle of enlarged arteries arises from the posterior cerebral branch of the basilar artery. The arrow points to early venous filling of the straight sinus. The frontal view (B) shows the midline location of this arteriovenous malformation.

For careful study of the cerebellopontine angle, *myeloencephalography* may be employed. This consists of the introduction of oily opaque contrast material into the lumbar subarachnoid space and its careful manipulation into the basilar cisterns and subsequently into the cerebellopontine angle. It is valuable for detailed study of eighth nerve tumors and arachnoiditis of this portion of the cerebral subarachnoid space.

The following are important considerations in the radiographic diagnosis of abnormalities of the brain. Signs and symptoms of the abnormalities discussed constitute indications for radiologic study.

Abnormal intracranial calcifications may be found in tumors, abscesses, hematomas, aneurysms, arteriovenous malformations, tuberculomas, tuberous sclerosis and toxoplasmosis. Displacement of normal midline calcifications, especially the partly calcified pineal body, indicates the presence of a space-taking lesion on the side opposite the displacement or, rarely, contraction of the brain on the side of the displacement.

Symmetrical enlargement of the cerebral ventricles suggests generalized brain atrophy or obstruction to the pathways of CSF circulation. The obstruction may be in the ventricular system or in the subarachnoid space and is usually due to tumor, inflammation or congenital anomaly. Displacement of the cerebral ventricles suggests a space-taking lesion on the side opposite the displacement or atrophy on the side to which the ventricles are displaced. The ventricles may also display abnormal contents, since an adjacent tumor may bulge into the lumen of the ventricles and be visible by virtue of air within the lumen.

Failure of certain intracranial arteries or veins to fill following appropriate injection of contrast material may have a number of causes. Normal variation may account for some of the curiosities, and one common finding is filling of both anterior cerebral arteries following injection on one side, there being no connection of the anterior cerebral arteries with the opposite side. Other causes of failure to fill the intracranial vasculature are spasm, thrombosis and generalized increased intracranial pressure.

Irregularity of the lumen of the intracranial arteries may be due to arteriosclerosis or arteritis. Intracranial vessels may be displaced to the opposite side in the presence of space-taking lesions, and other characteristic displacements may indicate the location of a mass within the cranium (elevation of the middle cerebral artery in temporal lobe lesions, for example).

The failure of intracranial arteries or veins to extend to the periphery suggests subdural hematoma, and if it is chronic, it may assume a lenticular shape which is quite characteristic (Figure 13). The filling of abnormal vessels with dense opacification and "staining" in the region of a vascular tumor may occur during the capillary phase, especially in meningiomas and glioblastomas (Figure 12). Individual vessels may be enlarged in aneurysms, certain tumors, and in arteriovenous malformations (Figure 14).

Other intracranial structures may show manifestations of abnormalities of the brain. Atrophy of the sella turcica with demineralization may be the consequence of increased intracranial pressure or an intrasellar tumor. Exaggerated convolutional impressions suggest increased intracranial pressure. Separation of skull sutures also suggests increased intracranial pressure, and this finding is practically confined to children. Finally, diffuse atrophy of the skull bones is another accompaniment of chronic increased intracranial pressure.

The Spinal Cord

Manifestations of abnormalities of the spinal cord may be detected on *plain films of the spine,* where erosion and deformity will be noted, or by *myelography,* using either opaque material or air.

On plain films of the spine, decreased intervertebral joint space suggests degenerative disc disease. An increase in the interpedicular distance on anteroposterior films suggests enlargement of the spinal cord resulting from syringomyelia or tumor. Vertebral erosion or enlargement of the intervertebral foramina suggest spinal cord or nerve root neoplasm, primary or metastatic.

Myelographic abnormalities provide important clues in the diagnosis of diseases of the spinal cord. A complete block may be found with herniated nucleus pulposus, neoplasm, arachnoiditis, or secondary to trauma. An extradural impression may be produced by a herniated disc, metastatic neoplasm, or abscess. An intradural deformity, ordinarily enlargement, suggests spinal cord or meningeal tumor, but arachnoiditis may produce bizarre intradural defects as well. An intramedullary deformity suggests syringomyelia or cord tumor. In some patients with herniated nucleus pulposus, the only myelographic manifestation may be a swollen nerve root or an asymmetrical root sleeve.

Selective arteriography of the arteries supplying the spinal cord has been employed to demonstrate the presence and extent of arteriovenous malformations. *Intraosseous venography* (injection into the spinous processes of several vertebrae) may opacify venous abnormalities in the spinal canal (varicosities, malformations).

Chapter 3

THE NOSE, THROAT, AND NECK

THE NOSE AND NASOPHARYNX

THE NASAL CAVITY and nasopharynx may be directly inspected visually, and there is thus little occasion for radiologic study. On occasion, film studies will provide confirmation of the clinical diagnosis and display in three dimensions and with more completeness the presence of an abnormality only suspected or seen incompletely by the usual speculum or mirror examination.

Two types of radiologic examination are employed, conventional frontal and lateral films and lateral fluoroscopy (and cinefluorography), with and without contrast material. Conventional frontal and lateral films show swelling of the mucous membrane, particularly that covering the nasal turbinates, in the presence of nasal infections, including the common cold, and in allergic states. Polyps and benign masses are seen as soft tissue filling defects in the nasal or nasopharyngeal airway (Figure 15), and

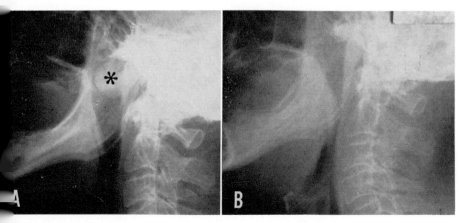

Figure 15. Carcinoma of the nasopharynx. The asterisk in A locates a rounded soft tissue mass protruding from the posterior wall of the nasopharynx. Biopsy proved this to be a carcinoma. Following radiation therapy the lesion disappeared (B).

31

malignant neoplasms have a similar appearance unless they erode and destroy bone, thereby affording a clue to the correct diagnosis. Enlargement of lymphoid tissue in the nasopharynx may encroach upon the airway; conversely, in children with immune deficiency states, the nasopharynx may be unusually spacious because of the lack of lymphoid tissue.

The instillation or insufflation of contrast material into the nose is ordinarily unnecessary and rarely employed for the better delineation of masses. It is of great value in establishing the diagnosis of choanal atresia, however. A soft catheter is introduced into the anterior aspect of the nasal cavity with the child in the supine position, and lateral films of the nose and nasopharynx are exposed with a horizontal x-ray beam following the introduction of opaque material. Complete obstructions are thus easily diagnosed, and the extent of incomplete obstructions may thereby be defined.

Vascular contrast studies are rarely indicated but may occasionally be of great value. The juvenile nasopharyngeal angiofibroma is a very vascular neoplasm, the identity and extent of which may be discovered by common or external carotid arteriography.

THE ORAL PHARYNX

Frontal and lateral conventional films and fluoroscopy and cinefluorography in the lateral position are also the methods of examination used for the oral pharynx. Standard film studies may disclose encroachments upon the proximal airway and food passages by lymphoid enlargements, tumors, or retropharyngeal abscesses or hematomas, and gross deformities of the soft palate and uvula may be found. Fluoroscopic examination offers the most versatility, however, permitting inspection of the mouth and pharynx during breathing, speaking and swallowing. Thus, the movements of the tongue and of the soft palate and uvula may be examined, and the movements of these parts during speech and swallowing may be studied. Particularly valuable is the use of lateral cinefluorography of the pharynx for the study of speech patterns and impediments. Simultaneously recording the sound of the patient's voice and the appearance of movements of the pharynx and mouth by lateral cinefluorography provides a combined record of considerable value to the speech therapist. The efficiency of the soft palate and uvula in preventing aspiration from the mouth into the nose during swallowing may be appraised by lateral cinefluorography during ingestion of a liquid barium-water mixture. Neuromuscular nasopharyngeal incoordination from any cause may prevent apposition of the uvula with the posterior pharyngeal wall during swallowing and allow retrograde aspiration of ingested material into the nasopharynx and nose.

THE LARYNX AND LARYNGEAL PHARYNX

The diagnostic work-up of a patient suspected of having disease of the larynx or adjacent structures includes a careful history and a physical examination dependent, for the most part, on indirect and direct visualization of the internal or mucosal aspect of the laryngeal apparatus. Radiologic examination may be added to this routine with ease, safety and profit. It has the advantage of pictorially displaying the entire larynx at rest and in motion and recording the findings on plain radiographs or on movie film so that they may be studied and reviewed by more than one observer and on more than one occasion. By radiologic means the larynx may be examined in coronal, sagittal and oblique planes and the findings transferred to a two-dimensional surface so that the relations between laryngeal structures distorted by disease are clearly depicted. Roentgenology of the larynx augments, confirms and supplements palpatory and laryngoscopic observations. In certain instances, it provides information obtainable in no other way, particularly regarding the subglottic space. Determination of the extent of laryngeal tumors and decisions regarding type of therapy to be employed are facilitated by roentgen examination.

Methods of Radiologic Examination

A variety of radiologic methods may be used to examine the larynx. Choice of which method or methods will be employed depends upon the kind of information to be obtained; time and facilities available; ability of the patient to cooperate; and the skill, experience and preference of the examiner.

Fluoroscopy, preferably with the image-amplified fluoroscope, provides useful information regarding the mobility of laryngeal structures. Changes in size, shape and position of the movable parts of the larynx are defined by contrast between the air-containing laryngeal chambers and the adjacent soft tissues. No opaque material need be used, but some experience is required in interpretation, since contrast is not great. Movements of the true vocal cords may be inspected with ease in this manner, and changes in the shape and volume of the laryngeal structures during the performance of various maneuvers may be seen. Examination during quiet respiration (or inspiration) and while phonating a high-pitched sound are the basic maneuvers employed. The examination may be permanently recorded on movie film (cinefluorography) and examined as often as desired. The examination may be preserved in this way for group viewing or for later consultation.

At the time of fluoroscopy, *fluoroscopic spot films* may be exposed to record findings. Four exposures will ordinarily suffice, PA views of the larynx in quiet respiration and during phonation and lateral views of the larynx under the same circumstances. If desired, certain other maneuvers may be employed, for example, the Valsalva maneuver, the Müller maneuver, and reverse phonation, to demonstrate specific areas to better advantage. By the use of spot films one may inexpensively and accurately record the gross morphology of the laryngeal structures and demonstrate evidence of normal or impaired mobility of the cords. Air within the pharynx, larynx and upper trachea provides negative contrast material without the necessity of utilizing an opaque medium. As with cinefluorography, contrast is not very great, and only grosser abnormalities are susceptible to careful examination in this way.

Conventional radiography in the lateral projection, using air as the naturally occurring negative contrast material, is the simplest means of obtaining radiologic information about the larynx. Exposures are ordinarily made in quiet respiration and during phonation. Such films show a true representation of laryngeal structures as seen from the side. The epiglottis stands out in relief against the air in the valleculae and in the pharynx. The aryepiglottic folds and the mucosa-covered arytenoids are well defined by surrounding air, and the laryngeal ventricles, ordinarily superimposed on each other, are seen as a cigar-shaped radiolucency near the lower margin of the thyroid cartilage. The true and false cords appear as bandlike soft tissue shadows above and below the ventricle. The anterior and posterior parts of the subglottic space are clearly seen on the lateral view. This lateral film is also valuable in examining the prelaryngeal soft tissues and the prevertebral space.

Detailed examination of the structure and function of the larynx may be obtained by *body section radiography*. The patient is examined in the coronal plane, ordinarily in the supine position. In this examination both the roentgen ray tube and the film beneath the patient move in opposite directions during an exposure lasting several seconds. This produces blurring of all structures anterior and posterior to the coronal plane of interest, this level being selected in advance by choosing an appropriate site above the table top to place the fulcrum of the lever arm that connects the tube and the film tray. This level may be varied in increments of 0.1 to 1.0 cm, thereby permitting step-by-step evaluation of successive coronal planes of the larynx from front to back. The examination is ordinarily performed both during phonation and quiet respiration. Utilizing air as the contrast agent, good visualization of the pyriform recesses, vestibule, true and false cords, laryngeal ventricle, and subglottic space can be obtained.

Positive contrast laryngography provides the most detailed radiographic information about the larynx. The technique utilizes a positive contrast agent which coats the mucosal surfaces of the larynx, producing sharp contrast between air in the laryngeal cavities and chambers and opaque material coating the walls. The pharynx and larynx are sprayed with a local anesthetic material, following which the opaque contrast agent is introduced in one of several ways. Utilizing a laryngeal mirror, the contrast material may be dripped through a curved needle directly into the larynx over the back of the tongue. Alternatively, the contrast agent may be sprayed into the oropharynx and aspirated into the larynx during deep breathing. A third method requires the passage of a soft rubber catheter through the glottis and into the upper trachea, at which point contrast material is deposited. The patient is then provoked to cough, and this activity distributes the contrast material throughout the larynx. The catheter is then removed.

Following the application of contrast material to the larynx, fluoroscopy, conventional or image-amplified, may be performed, and cinefluorography may be done. Fluoroscopic spot films may be made, and conventional frontal and lateral roentgen exposures may be utilized. Body section radiography may also be employed but is seldom necessary. The films are made in the frontal and lateral projections during quiet respiration; phonation; the Valsalva and Müller maneuvers, if desired; reverse phonation; and sometimes at the height of swallowing. This latter maneuver elevates the larynx and exposes to view a portion of the trachea which might otherwise be hidden by the clavicle and other structures in the vicinity of the superior thoracic aperture.

Atropine or some other parasympatholytic agent is commonly given as premedication in order to render the mucous membrane of the larynx dry so that the contrast material will adhere. Many iodinated opaque materials have been utilized; oily Dionosil® is safe and effective. If the examination is properly performed, contrast material will be seen to line the pyriform recesses and vestibule, to coat the false and true vocal cords, and to extend into the laryngeal ventricles on both sides. The subglottic space will be well seen in both frontal and lateral views, and the mucous membrane covering the arytenoids and aryepiglottic folds will be thrown into bold relief in the lateral projection.

Radiologic Reflections of Pathologic Alterations

CHANGES IN SIZE. Increase in the size of laryngeal structures commonly indicates the presence of an abnormality. The epiglottis, as seen in the lateral view defined by air in the valleculae anteriorly and in the pharynx posteriorly, may be considerably increased in size because of inflammation. Epiglottitis may produce enlargement by swelling of the covering mucous membrane resulting from edema in allergic states or a combination of edema and cellular infiltration in inflammatory or infectious lesions. Neoplasms of the epiglottis produce irregular and usually asymmetrical enlargement. The increase in size may be so marked as to encroach upon the upper laryngeal airway and produce respiratory difficulty. Similarly, inflammation and neoplasms of the true and false vocal cords may produce increase in size of these structures. Laryngitis commonly produces symmetrical enlargement of the true cords and may interfere markedly with their mobility, with resultant hoarseness. Benign neoplasms may present as localized nodular enlargements of the cords, usually unilateral, projecting into the adjacent airway. Carcinomas of the true cords produce irregular asymmetrical enlargement and may result in fixation. Some degree of inflammatory infiltration and edema accompany malignant neoplasms of the true cords, and to a varying extent the enlargement of these structures is due to edema. Hazy loss of the normally clean-cut horizontal air shadow just below the true vocal cords commonly accompanies both inflammatory swelling and neoplastic invasion.

Increase in size of the soft tissue spaces between air-containing structures may also be seen in the larynx, usually secondary to a malignant neoplasm. Increase in the width of the soft tissue space between air in the laryngeal vestibule and air in one of the pyriform sinuses may result from infiltration of this area by a malignant neoplasm arising in the vicinity. Similarly, the prelaryngeal and retrolaryngeal soft tissue spaces may be increased in anteroposterior diameter by contiguous spread of a neoplasm.

Pathologic enlargement of the laryngeal ventricle is referred to as laryngocele. The dilated ventricle may lie entirely within the larynx and displace the false cord upward and medially, so-called internal laryngocele. It may, however, enlarge in a tubular fashion superiorly and laterally, finally to penetrate the posterior part of the thyrohyoid membrane and appear as an abnormal gas-containing structure in the upper part of the neck (an external laryngocele) in the vicinity of the hyoid bone. Any maneuver which tends to balloon the ventricles will be helpful in demonstrating such an abnormality (modified Valsalva maneuver and reverse phonation, for example). Body section radiography in the frontal plane will display the anatomy to good advantage, and the rhythmic distention of the laryngocele may be shown by cinefluorography.

Decrease in size of the laryngeal airway is usually the result of enlargement, symmetrical or otherwise, of the adjacent soft tissues or cartilages (Figure 16). Carcinoma of the pyriform recess may produce irregular narrowing of the air column within the recess, and a neoplasm of the true cords or one involving

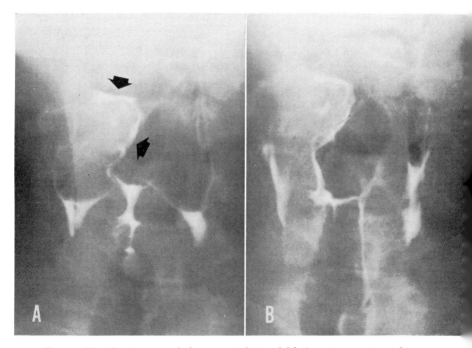

Figure 16. Carcinoma of the aryepiglottic fold (positive contrast laryngogram). The mucosal surfaces of the larynx are coated with contrast material which renders them opaque. The arrows in A point to a sizable mass arising from the right aryepiglottic fold and projecting into the laryngeal vestibule. This film was made during reverse phonation, and as a consequence the pyriform sinuses are distended. The true and false cords are outlined on their medial aspects. In B the tumor is again seen, but this film was exposed during inspiration, and the pyriform recesses are no longer distended. The true and false cords are retracted laterally, and the airway is unobstructed.

the subglottic space will produce irregular decrease in size of the airway adjacent to these structures. Inflammatory, infectious or traumatic edema of the laryngeal structures may produce marked narrowing of the airway with wheezing respirations and stridor. The laryngeal ventricles may be markedly decreased in size or even obliterated by swelling or other enlargement of the adjacent true or false cords. These ventricles are seen so consistently on lateral films of the neck exposed during phonation that one should strongly suspect infection, faulty innervation or new growth if they are not visualized.

CHANGES IN SHAPE AND POSITION. The normally smooth contours of the mucosa-covered surfaces of the larynx may be distorted by irregular new growths, and their shape may be altered by swelling resulting from any cause. Particularly notable are changes in the position of some of the soft parts of the larynx secondary to vocal cord paralysis. The paralyzed cord may be slightly elevated, and the ventricle is commonly wider on the paralyzed side. During phonation the two true cords appose normally in the midline, and no abnormality may be seen, though a slight fullness in the subglottic area may be noted on the paralyzed side, on which side the tip of the pyriform recess may be slightly elevated. However, during quiet respiration, the affected cord does not retract normally along the lateral laryngeal wall, projecting instead into the lumen of the airway, and the ventricle on the affected side gapes widely and appears much larger than the thin slit ordinarily seen in this view during quiet respiration. Failure of the true cord to relax is due to paralysis of the vocalis muscle, the function of which is to release tension on the vocal ligament.

The shape of the laryngeal airway may be markedly altered by abnormalities in the soft tissues forming the walls of these air-containing cavities. The airway may be encroached upon by swellings of whatever cause, in which case the deformity is often symmetrical. Tumors of the soft parts commonly encroach irregularly and asymmetrically upon the airway. Certain inflammatory lesions are prone to produce laryngeal stenosis, particularly diphtheria and tuberculosis, in which case the airway may end abruptly where fusion of the soft parts has occurred, often at the level of the junction of the cricoid cartilage with the upper trachea. A characteristic deformity of the air shadow may thus be produced: the air column is funnel-shaped, with the apex of the funnel pointing inferiorly.

From the radiologic aspect, stridor can be produced almost everywhere in the larynx by bulky parts or protruding or redundant folds without extralaryngeal pathology, and if one suspects such a possibility, the roentgen diagnosis usually can be made. The airway is narrowed, and the soft parts are deformed by projecting into the lumen, depending upon what part of the larynx is involved. In infants and children excessive folding of the epiglottis with shortening of the aryepiglottic folds is a common cause. This is usually associated with some degree of flabbiness of the mesenchymal tissue of the larynx, and the poorly supported epiglottis may flutter over the superior laryngeal aperture, partly obstructing it during inspiration. Tracheomalacia producing obstructive symptoms during expiration may also occur in infancy. Image-amplified fluoroscopy and cinefluorography in the lateral projection will demonstrate the abnormality.

The laryngeal cartilages may be the site of origin of benign tumors (chondromas) which project into the airway and alter the shape and position of normal structures. Such tumors commonly arise from the cricoid cartilage and may show calcific mottling, vague trabeculation, and stippled or irregular amorphous calcification. The laryngeal cartilages may be destroyed by invading carcinoma from adjacent structures, and if they are calcified, this destruction may be obvious radiologically. Great caution should be exercised, however, in diagnosing malignant destruction of laryngeal cartilages, since calcification within them is extremely irregular and unpredictable. Calcified laryngeal cartilages may also occasionally be deformed by fracture, though this is uncommon and difficult to diagnose radiologically.

CHANGES IN MOBILITY. The three most common causes of loss of or decrease in mobility of the laryngeal structures are edema, carcinoma and recurrent nerve palsy. The portions of the larynx affected by an infiltrating malignant neoplasm may be fixed and immovable, and their failure to move normally may be displayed accurately at fluoroscopy and recorded by cinefluorography. Fixation of movable laryngeal structures is rarely produced by edema, though considerable decrease in normal mobility may result. Vocal cord paralysis results in a relatively immobile true cord projecting into the laryngeal airway and failing to retract during quiet respiration. Anteroposterior fluoroscopic spot films made during quiet respiration and during phonation will accurately document this abnormality. It may be shown more elegantly by body section radiography and positive contrast laryngography. Failure of the epiglottis and aryepiglottic folds to close the superior laryngeal aperture, resulting in aspiration, may be demonstrated by barium swallow in the lateral projection. This is best recorded by cinefluorography.

FOREIGN BODIES. Impaction of a sizeable foreign body in the larynx may produce suffocation and sudden death, commonly while eating. However, foreign bodies rarely lodge in the larynx otherwise, and the most common location for foreign bodies in the vicinity is in the retrolaryngeal soft tissues. They reach this location after being swallowed, and fishbones are common offenders. They may lodge in the laryngeal pharynx and produce adjacent soft tissue swelling. Lateral films made with careful technique may show an opaque foreign body. The diagnostic problem more commonly presents in a different way, however. Because of the irregular calcification of the laryngeal cartilages, there is a tendency to overdiagnose retrolaryngeal opaque foreign bodies in patients with history, symptoms and findings compatibile with the diagnosis. Thinly calcified posterior portions of the thyroid cartilage, the posterior lamina of the cricoid cartilage, the faintly and irregularly calcified arytenoid cartilages, and the occasionally calcified triticeous cartilage may mimic retrolaryngeal foreign bodies. Foreign bodies lodging in the region of the larynx may be a genuine problem in the postlaryngectomy patient where the food passage in the vicinity of the operative site may be tented and deformed, providing a pocket wherein poorly chewed foreign materials may lodge.

RETROLARYNGEAL MASSES. These may be inflammatory (abcess), neoplastic or traumatic (hematoma) in origin. The anteroposterior diameter of the postcricoid space in the adult is equal to about 0.7 times the anteroposterior dimension of the body of the fourth cervical vertebra in the male (0.6 in the female). A retrolaryngeal mass displaces the air passage anteriorly and increases the thickness of the postcricoid space. In infants and small children it is important to remember that the prevertebral soft tissues may appear thickened if the lateral film is exposed with the neck in flexion or in the expiratory phase of respiration. In both cases the appearance of an apparent retrolaryngeal mass is caused by anterior buckling of the trachea. Suspicion of bona fide anterior displacement of the airway by a retrolaryngeal tumefaction should be aroused if the larynx and trachea are dislocated anteriorly and the trachea is not buckled.

Radiologic examination of the larynx may be profitably employed to augment, confirm and complement other means of physical examination, particularly laryngoscopy. Properly employed, the radiologic examination does not compete with other means of study but provides additional information and occasionally discloses abnormalities with a certainty unobtainable by other methods. It is especially valuable in permitting the examiner to inspect the larynx in its entirety, thereby facilitating comparisons between symmetrical parts and exposing the interrelations of the laryngeal structures to careful study. Radiologic examination of the larynx should be performed prior to biopsy, since operative procedures produce edema and distortion of laryngeal structures.

Choice of radiologic method of examination depends upon the information needed or desired. The search for foreign bodies, for epiglottic enlargement or irregularity, and for anterior subglottic disease is best accomplished on simple lateral films of the larynx. Vocal cord paralysis may be established by exposing fluoroscopic spot films in the coronal plane in quiet respiration and during phonation. Laryngeal carcinoma is best studied in frontal and lateral planes either by body section radiography or positive contrast laryngography. Mobility of laryngeal structures is most satisfactorily examined by image-amplified fluoroscopy and displayed by cinefluorography.

Radiologic study of the larynx may be expected to provide useful information, provided that reasonable care is taken in selecting the proper examination and in its performance. Risk and discomfort to the patient are slight, and the examination may be performed with a minimum of time and inconvenience.

THE NECK

Abnormalities of the other soft tissues of the neck may at times be detected roentgenologically, but the manifestations are usually nonspecific.

Thyroid enlargement may be seen as a soft tissue swelling, if large enough, and tumors of the thyroid commonly displace the trachea. Calcifications may be found in both benign and malignant thyroid tumors on conventional films. Methods have been developed to selectively opacify the arteries to the thyroid, but general clinical applicability has yet to be established. Direct injection of diffusable contrast material into the thyroid gland is in the experimental stage.

Enlargement of the parathyroid glands is rarely detected on conventional films. If the lesion is large enough, it may slightly displace the barium-opacified esophagus.

A variety of congenital and acquired cysts may be seen as soft tissue masses on films of the neck (lymphangioma, branchial cleft and thyroglossal duct cysts, for example). Some may be aspirated, and following this, contrast material may be injected to define, roentgenographically, their size, shape and extent (rarely done). Fistulas to the surface of the skin of the neck may require contrast injection to demonstrate their course and ramifications prior to surgical therapy.

Roentgen study of the salivary glands may at times be valuable. Conventional films may show opaque calculi within the ducts of the salivary glands and occasionally within the glands themselves. Opacification of the ducts and acini of the glands with contrast material is required for careful radiologic study. Nonopaque stones, sialectasis, strictures, masses, abscesses and diffuse infiltrative processes may be demonstrated. Some abnormalities have specific sialographic appearances (Sjogren's syndrome, for example).

Other neck masses, including metastases to lymph nodes, may show as soft tissue opacities on films of the neck, but usually these are better studied by palpation and perhaps by biopsy.

Chapter 4

THE LUNGS

ORDINARY CHEST FILMS

THE ROUTINE VIEWS of the chest exposed for study of the lungs are the erect posteroanterior and lateral films made at a target-to-film distance of six feet. Such films are ordinarily exposed in moderate to deep inspiration, but that is sometimes not controllable, particulary in small infants. No preparation of the patient is necessary, and if he is able to sit or stand, there are no important contraindications. Indeed, chest films are often exposed periodically in asymptomatic healthy people as a screening test for smoldering or incipient pulmonary disease, particularly in susceptible populations or in persons regularly exposed to pulmonary inflammatory disease, such as those who work in and about hospitals.

The lungs are examined for contour, expansion and clarity. The following are kinds of abnormalities susceptible to display on ordinary chest films, suspicion of which constitutes the usual indication for the examination.

Pulmonary *infi'trations* manifest themselves radiologically as areas of increased density within the otherwise radiolucent lung parenchyma, the pathological equivalent of which is the presence of abnormal material of some sort in the alveoli or the interstitial tissues. The prototype of this kind of abnormality is bacterial pneumonia, where the abnormal material consists of edema fluid, microorganisms and leukocytes, in addition to which there may be pus, depending upon the type and virulence of the organisms. Thickening of the interstitial tissues ordinarily presents a more linear and radial pattern and may be the result of fibrosis, edema, cellular infiltration or a combination of these. Interstitial pulmonary infiltrations are common in asthma, emphysema, collagen diseases, pneumoconioses, viral infections and the nonspecific

44

fibrosis associated with aging. Alveolar infiltrations commonly have a fluffier appearance presenting as few or many ill-defined and poorly circumscribed opacities. Pulmonary edema and acute bacterial pneumonia are examples of conditions which may produce acute disseminated alveolar infiltrations. Chronic disseminated alveolar infiltrative disease has many causes, the most common of which are the following: granulomatous pulmonary infection, particularly tuberculosis; alveolar cell carcinoma; sarcoidosis; pulmonary alveolar proteinosis; pulmonary hemosiderosis; lymphoma; and pulmonary alveolar microlithiasis.

Consolidation of all or part of the lung is ordinarily easily detected on routine chest films because it presents a more dense and confluent density than the usual infiltration. Branching radiolucencies representing air in patent bronchi may be seen within the lesion ("air bronchogram"). Solidification of a part of the lung is the pathologic change represented on chest films by a more or less solid density called consolidation, and its common causes are lobar or lobular pneumonia (Figure 17) and infarction.

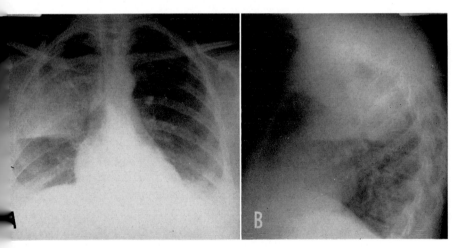

Figure 17. Lobar pneumonia. The anterior segment of the right upper lobe is densely and homogeneously consolidated (pneumococcal pneumonia). The straight inferior border (A) is produced by the minor fissure which separates the anterior segment of the upper lobe from the middle lobe. The lateral view (B) shows the consolidated portion of the upper lobe.

Masses in the lung are usually due to replacement of pulmonary tissue by an enlarging neoplasm or sharply demarcated inflammatory process. They appear as dense, often lobulated, sometimes multiple, homogeneous soft tissue densities located within the parenchyma peripherally or near the lung hilus. A solitary nodular pulmonary lesion is most likely a carcinoma, granuloma or hamartoma. Multiple pulmonary masses commonly represent metastases to the lung or pleura (Figure 18) but may be seen in pleural mesotheliomas. Masses which cavitate are usually inflammatory, but about 10 percent of carcinomas of the lung contain cavities. Calcified pulmonary lesions are almost alway benign. Masses may protrude into the lung from the pleura, ribs, intercostal muscles, nerves and blood vessels or from the heart, great vessels or other mediastinal structures. For this reason it is often necessary to obtain multiple views in many projections or even unusual and special views in order to determine whether or not the lesion is pulmonary or arises from structures adjacent to the lung. Masses within the lung will ordinarily prove to be malignant neoplasms or granulomatous infection, though at times unresolved pneumonia resulting from bacteria may produce an appearance indistinguishable from a mass, as may oil aspiration pneumonia. Finally, loculated interlobar pleural fluid may give the appearance of a "pseudo-tumor."

Atelectasis is demonstrable radiologically on ordinary posteroanterior and lateral chest films as a usually homogeneous area of pulmonary opacification, with relatively smooth margins and with evidence of loss of functioning lung volume (Figure 19). If the involved lung, lobe or segment is completely collapsed, diagnosis may be simple, but partial atelectasis may be difficult to identify. Secondary signs which are useful include shift of a fissure line, shift of the hilus or mediastinum, elevation of the diaphragm on the affected side, and crowding of the ribs on the involved side. Compensatory emphysema in the uninvolved lobe or segments may also help in the diagnosis. Atelectasis may rarely be due to compression but will usually be the result of bronchial obstruction from a tumor, inflammatory products or effects, or a foreign body. Unless the cause is obvious, special views or procedures, particularly bronchography, may be indicated.

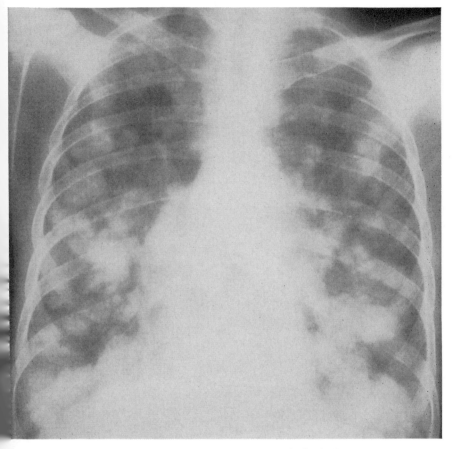

Figure 18. Pulmonary metastases (carcinoma of the kidney). The lungs are filled with large and small nodular lesions due to hematogenous spread from hypernephroma. The radiographic diagnosis is based upon the fact that the lesions are multiple, of different sizes, are discrete and well defined and do not, at this stage, impair the ability of the patient to take a deep breath.

Overinflation of all or part of the lung (*emphysema*) may be atrophic or obstructive. The atrophic type is usually generalized, and x-ray films show only diminished number and size of bronchovascular markings per unit volume of lung, without marked evidence of overinflation. Obstructive emphysema may be generalized as a result of diffuse obstructive changes in the terminal bronchioles or localized as a result of an obstructing lesion in one

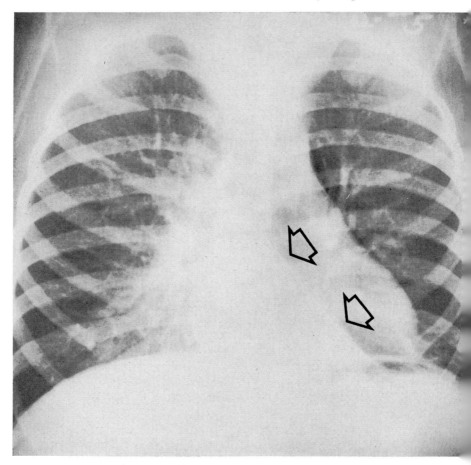

Figure 19. Left lower lobe atelectasis. Collapse of the left lower lobe is responsible for the dense triangular opacity behind the heart (arrows). Compensatory emphysema of the left upper lobe accounts for the radiolucency which occupies the left hemithorax, but the number of vascular markings in the left lung is smaller than normal when compared with the right. In addition, the left hilus is lower than the right, a finding suggestive of left lower lobe atelectasis and the opposite of the normal condition.

of the bronchi (segmental emphysema may be an early sign of carcinoma of the lung). In obstructive emphysema the volume of the affected part is increased, and secondary signs of the same may be seen on ordinary chest films. These include flattening and depression of the diaphragm, shift of a hilus or of the mediastinum, increased diameter of the thorax, and spreading of the ribs. In addition, the heart may seem small and the pulmonary arteries in the hilus may appear unusually prominent. Obstructive emphysema resulting from diffuse bronchiolar disease is much more common than that resulting from localized obstruction of a bronchus secondary to such things as infection and neoplasm.

Pneumothorax is usually clearly displayed on ordinary chest films if sufficient air escapes into the pleural space, and the lack of vascular and bronchopulmonary markings in the involved area may be obvious. If it is a tension pneumothorax, the mediastinum will be shifted to the opposite side. If it is accompanied by fluid in the pleural space, then a distinct horizontal air-fluid level will be seen on films made with a horizontal x-ray beam such as routine erect PA and lateral chest films. If the amount of air in the pleural space is small, then special maneuvers may be necessary to display the altered anatomy. A film made in expiration may show a pneumothorax better than the usual inspiratory film. Pneumothorax may be traumatic or spontaneous resulting from rupture of a subpleural emphysematous bleb, or it may be chronic resulting from bronchopleural fistula from any cause.

Pleural effusion is seen as a homogeneous opacity obscuring the lungs and separating them from the ribs (Figure 20). If free, the fluid will settle to the most dependent part of the thorax. On ordinary erect posteroanterior and lateral chest films, fluid in the pleural space will be seen posteriorly and laterally causing blunting and then obliteration of the posterior and lateral costophrenic gutters or angles. Special views, particularly decubitus views, may be necessary to demonstrate with certainty the presence of fluid in the pleural space. If loculated or unusually thick (like clotted blood), the fluid may fail to shift with a shift in position of the patient and may present an appearance more like a mass than free fluid. The causes of fluid in the pleural space are very numerous, but most will be found associated with pulmonary or pleural infections, neoplasms, infarction or trauma.

SPECIAL VIEWS

Oblique views of the chest are routinely used in the evaluation of the shape of the heart. They frequently have value as well in examination of abnormalities of the lungs. Rib erosion from

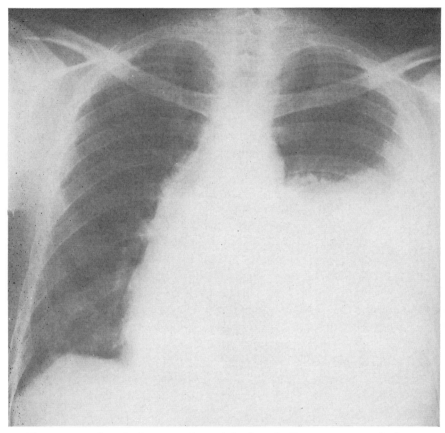

Figure 20. Pleural effusion. A huge left pleural effusion occupies the lower two thirds of the left hemithorax and has displaced the heart and mediastinal structures somewhat to the right. A small amount of fluid has crept into the upper lateral part of the pleural space, producing a rounded upper margin to the effusion and obliterating the usually sharp costophrenic angle.. The upper margin of the pleural effusion is rounded because of the meniscus effect produced by wetting of the superior part of the lateral pleural wall.

an adjacent malignant neoplasm may be visible only on oblique views or be better shown by them. Localization of a lesion to a particular part of the lung may require oblique film studies, and the relations between pulmonary lesions and adjacent mediastinal or bony structures may be best displayed in that way. It is usual to obtain posteroanterior and lateral chest films first and then determine whether or not additional views are necessary and if so, which ones. *Lordotic films* are of particular value in suspected or actual lesions of the apices of the lungs. By tilting the patient for the lordotic view, the clavicles are elevated away from the lungs and the apices more satisfactorily exposed. This view may be of special value in the study of patients with pulmonary tuberculosis and is often used routinely as part of the follow-up film examination. At times, cavities not seen on ordinary or oblique films may be visible on the lordotic view (Figure 21).

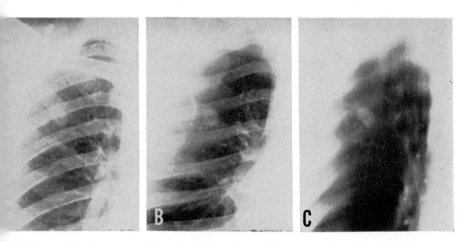

Figure 21. Cavitary pulmonary tuberculosis (three views). In A, the right upper lung in a standard posteroanterior projection, one sees an area of infiltration with a central radiolucency. The lordotic view, B, shows the lesion from a slightly different point of view and emphasizes the presence of the cavity within it. Body section radiography, C, blurs the structures in front of and behind the lesion, mostly the ribs, allowing the area of infiltration and central cavitation to be seen without distractions.

Films exposed in *inspiration and expiration* will demonstrate the mobility of the diaphragm without the need for fluoroscopy. Such films are also indicated and valuable in the study of patients suspected of having aspirated a foreign body with subsequent development of atelectasis or emphysema. A small pneumothorax may be best shown on expiratory chest films, and the degree of pulmonary compliance may be grossly estimated from the ability of the lungs to expand and contract.

At times, *overpenetrated views*, such as those obtained with the Potter-Bucky diaphragm, are necessary for adequate evaluation of the chest. That is particularly so in a very large or obese patient or when great cardiomegaly impairs the examiner's ability to see the left lower lung. The search for calcium within pulmonary mass lesions may require overpenetrated views, as may the demonstration of rib erosion or destruction from inflammatory or neoplastic disease in the lungs. Hiatus hernias may manifest themselves as soft tissue opacities containing an air fluid level located behind the heart on overpenetrated frontal films of the chest. The lateral film will ordinarily accurately display the abnormality as well.

Decubitus views of the chest are made with a horizontal x-ray beam and with the patient lying on one or the other side. Such a position will cause overexpansion of the uppermost lung, since expansion of the lowermost lung is impeded by the patient's posture. Such a film may display to better advantage a lesion in the lung which is overexpanded or eliminate densities produced by platelike atelectasis on the ordinary PA film. Decubitus views are utilized most often to demonstrate shifts of fluid in the pleural space, thereby confirming that an opacity in the chest represents pleural effusion. At times that is unnecessary, but it is particularly indicated when the distinction between an elevated hemidiaphragm and an infrapulmonary effusion is difficult. If an effusion is present and if the fluid is free to move in the pleural space, the decubitus film will demonstrate layering of the fluid along the dependent lateral chest wall. At times the decubitus views are valuable in demonstrating shifts of opacities within pulmonary lesions themselves. In particular, the demonstration of change in position of a nodule within a cavity, indicating that the nodule lies free within the cavity, suggests the diagnosis of intracavity pulmonary fungus ball (aspergilloma).

Fluoroscopy of the chest is rarely performed and is useful mainly for appraisal of diaphragmatic movements. It will also show the curious mediastinal shift and swing during inspiration and expiration in a patient with an obstructed bronchus resulting from aspirated foreign body, but plain films will disclose the same abnormality. The relationships between intrathoracic structures may be well displayed by fluoroscopy, and at times the patient may be examined in this way to determine the best projection for exposing permanent films. Fluoroscopy may be of particular value in localizing a lesion difficult to see on the lateral film prior to performing body section radiography. Except for permanently recording mediastinal or diaphragmatic movement or for bronchography, cinefluorography has little use in the examination of the lungs.

Body section radiography is especially valuable in the study of lesions of the lungs suspected to contain calcium or a cavity (Figure 21). Unequivocal demonstration of the presence of either cavitation or calcification within a lesion strongly suggests that the lesion is benign and inflammatory, though that is not always the case (hamartomas calcify and some carcinomas cavitate). Body section radiography may also be valuable in searching for tiny metastases in the lungs which are not visible on ordinary films, though in that instance one must make very many "cuts" of both lungs in order to maximize the possibility of finding small lesions. The shape of a pulmonary lesion which borders on the hilus may be better shown by body section radiography, and at times one can demonstrate bronchial deformity or obstruction in this way and thus explain the pathogenesis and even the etiology of the pulmonary lesion.

Recumbent films of the chest are exposed when the patient is unable to stand or sit and are likely to be less satisfactory than films made in the erect position. Pulmonary expansion is less than optimum with the patient in the recumbent position, and the short x-ray tube-to-film distance necessitated by the recumbent position produces some unsharpness of detail. *Portable films* of the chest exposed with modern equipment may be quite satisfactory but are no substitute for films exposed in the Radiology Department.

BRONCHOGRAPHY

The contrast material may be introduced into the tracheobronchial tree in a number of ways, including transtracheal catheterization by the Seldinger technique used for arterial catheterization. A variety of contrast materials has been employed, including barium, and if the patient is able to cough effectively, it is unlikely that barium in the tracheobronchial tree will cause any permanent difficulty. It is inert and probably less damaging to the bronchial mucosa than aqueous iodinated contrast substances. The oily opaques are ideal.

Bronchography is indicated in a patient with symptoms of bronchopulmonary disease in whom chest films fail to demonstrate adequately the pathologic anatomy or when ordinary films suggest a diagnosis which must be confirmed by opacification of the tracheobronchial tree. Examples of such abnormalities follow.

Intrinsic abnormalities which are best displayed by bronchography are of several types. Congenital anomalies of origin and distribution of the bronchi are ordinarily easily shown. Bronchi do not ordinarily communicate with an area of bronchopulmonary sequestration. Inflammatory tracheal and bronchial lesions are a common indication for bronchography. Bronchitis is manifested as mucosal irregularities, while bronchiectasis is seen as fusiform or saccular bronchial dilatations in which contrast material pools and which may even contain fluid levels if the cavities are large enough (Figure 22). Bronchography is of critical importance in the preoperative evaluation of patients with bronchiectasis, since the surgeon will wish to remove all of the involved segments if possible and feasible. Bronchial strictures resulting from inflammatory disease of the epithelium and perhaps associated with obstructive emphysema or atelectatsis may be displayed bronchographically, as may the presence of foreign bodies or granulomas within the lumen which may distort or obstruct the airway. Bronchopleural fistulas may allow the passage of contrast material from the bronchi into the pleural space, and other curious fistulas which are much rarer (such as bronchorenal) may also be shown in this way.

Neoplastic pulmonary lesions may be studied with profit by bronchography, and at times bronchography will be required to differentiate an area of chronic or unresolved pneumonia from a pulmonary neoplasm. Bronchi are commonly patent in an area of pneumonia, while malignant neoplasms tend to obstruct bronchi early, producing areas of obstructive atelectasis, emphysema or pneumonitis distal to the lesion.

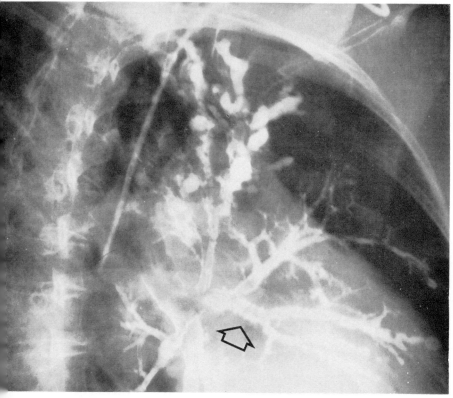

Figure 22. Bronchitis and bronchiectasis (bronchogram). Cylindrical and saccular dilatation of the bronchi is evident in the upper lung following filling of the bronchial tree with an opaque contrast substance. In addition, the irregularities in the mucosal surface to which the arrow points are produced by dilated bronchial glands and indicate the presence of pronounced chronic bronchitis.

Bronchography may also be of value in the study of abnormalities of expansion, both atelectasis and emphysema, though most often the study is indicated in a patient suspected of having localized disease resulting from inflammation, neoplasm or foreign body. Extrinsic abnormalities which displace the trachea and bronchi may also be readily demonstrated by opacification of the airway, but such an examination is not often indicated or necessary. Lesions of the pleura, such as large mesotheliomas, and lesions of the thoracic spine and rib cage, such as large chondromas or chondrosarcomas, may produce deformities of the tracheobronchial tree. Lesions of the diaphragm, such as tumors, primary or metastatic, and diaphragmatic defects permitting herniation of abdominal contents into the thorax, may displace the trachea and bronchi, but unless massive, bronchography is rarely necessary to define the pathologic changes present. Abnormalities of the heart and great vessels, such as gross cardiac enlargement (particularly left atrial enlargement), tumors, or aneurysms may produce tracheal and bronchial deformations or even extrinsic obstruction of accessible parts of the airway. Finally, inflammatory and neoplastic lesions of adjacent structures may deform or even invade the trachea or bronchi from without, such abnormalities as suppurating hilar lymph nodes or carcinoma of the esophagus.

PULMONARY ANGIOGRAPHY

The pulmonary vascularity may be opacified following intravenous injection of contrast material or, more adequately, by selective pulmonary arteriography. The kinds of abnormalities which are susceptible to display by pulmonary angiography, suspicion of which constitute indications for the procedure, include the following.

Vascular lesions in the lungs are best displayed in this way. Such lesions include pulmonary arteriovenous fistulas and pulmonary varicosities. Pulmonary thromboemboli are seen as filling defects in the pulmonary artery and its branches by contrast angiography, and such a procedure may help to explain the presence of pulmonary opacities resulting from infarction. It must be remembered, however, that most pulmonary emboli do not produce infarction. Peripheral pulmonary artery coarctations which produce curious flame-shaped densities may be seen angiographically, and anomalies of and obstruction to venous return are well shown in this way, particularly if the injection of contrast agent is made selectively into the main pulmonary artery.

Parenchymal pulmonary lesions which are seen on ordinary chest films as nonspecific opacities may provide indication for pulmonary angiography when distinction between pneumonia, neoplasm and infarction is necessary. The pulmonary artery branches in an area involved by pneumonia are patent and not grossly abnormal, while the vessels to an infarcted area are often seen to be obstructed. Pulmonary artery branches in an area occupied by a malignant neoplasm are similarly obstructed, though they may only be encased and distorted and occasionally only displaced. In regard to malignant disease, pulmonary angiography has its greatest value in neoplasms adjacent to the hilus or mediastinum which may be assumed to be unresectable if they have invaded or obstructed one of the main pulmonary arteries (Figure 23).

BRONCHIAL ARTERIOGRAPHY

Using special catheters usually introduced percutaneously into a femoral artery, one or both bronchial arteries may be selectively catheterized, followed by injection of small amounts of contrast material and serial filming. The examination has been suggested as valuable in the differentiation of a benign from a malignant neoplasm and in the differential diagnosis of pneumonia and neoplasm. While it is true that some malignant tumors have characteristic vascular patterns, some areas of intense inflammation will also show increased vascularity, and the differentiation may be difficult. As a clinical procedure with therapeutic or prognostic implications, it is of limited value.

DIAGNOSTIC PNEUMOTHORAX

Pneumothorax as a diagnostic procedure is rarely employed. It may be useful in demonstrating that an intrathoracic lesion arises from the pleura rather than from the lung, and it may demonstrate the effects of adhesions obliterating all or part of the pleural space.

PERCUTANEOUS NEEDLE BIOPSY
OF PULMONARY LESIONS

This procedure may be performed by radiologist or surgeon, though it is often done in concert, the surgeon placing the needle while the radiologist exercises fluoroscopic control and guidance. By this technique small amounts of tissue may be removed for microscopic examination and allow the establishment of a correct diagnosis short of thoracotomy. It is particularly useful in solid lesions adjacent to the pleura, but lesions more deeply placed may at times be successfully needled. It also has value in the diagnosis of disseminated pulmonary disease, though on such occasions a "little" thoracotomy with removal of slightly more tissue under direct vision may be preferable.

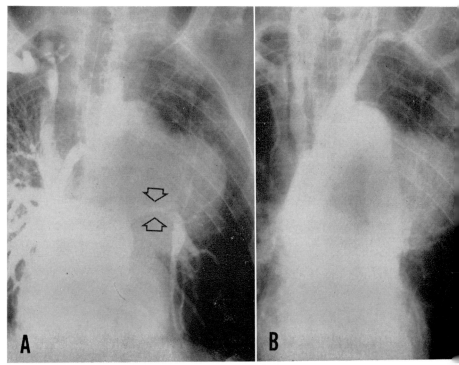

Figure 23. Carcinoma of the lung (angiogram). Contrast material was injected intravenously into the right upper extremity. Serial filming was carried out, and in A one sees a pulmonary arteriogram. The arrows point to the markedly narrowed left pulmonary artery. It has been encircled and encased by the very large left hilar mass which proved to be a broncho-genic carcinoma. The blood supply to the left lung is markedly reduced because of the invasion of the left pulmonary artery. In B, a later film from the serial sequence, the descending aorta can be seen to course pos-terior to the mass. There is no evidence of dilatation of the aorta or irregu-larity of its wall to suggest that the sizable soft tissue lesion is an aneu-rysm.

Chapter 5

THE MEDIASTINUM

PLAIN FILMS

THE RADIOLOGIC EXPRESSION of mediastinal disease is usually an abnormality in the size or shape of the mediastinum as seen on plain films. The *routine posteroanterior and lateral views* made in the erect position may offer important clues to the diagnosis and are the first studies indicated when mediastinal abnormalities are suspected. Tumors which deform the mediastinum and partially replace or displace its contents may be localized on frontal and lateral films, allowing preliminary speculation as to their type (Figure 24). Air-fluid levels may suggest the presence

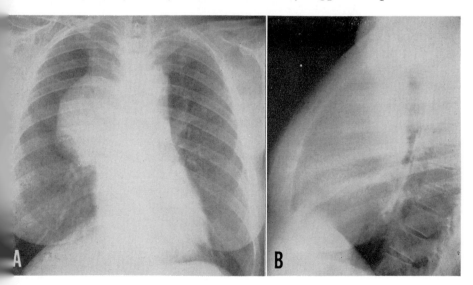

Figure 24. Thymoma. (A) The posteroanterior chest film shows a sizable soft tissue mass projecting from the mediastinum toward the right side. (B) The lateral film reveals the mass to be located anteriorly. No calcification is seen. Such anterior mediastinal masses commonly prove to be thymomas, teratomas or substernal thyroids.

of an abscess or necrotic neoplasm or the need for barium studies of the esophagus. Abnormal bulges and deformities may be due to curious malformations of the heart or lesions of the pericardium, and aneurysms or poststenotic vascular enlargments may mimic mediastinal tumors. Posteroanterior and lateral films will generally suggest the need for other special views which will more completely expose the contours of the suspected abnormality.

There are many *special views* of the mediastinum which are valuable in the search for abnormalities. Oblique views are especially helpful for localizing mass lesions, and sometimes views with only slight obliquity may be more valuable than the routine oblique studies. Lordotic films allow visualization of the lateral contours of lesions in the superior mediastinum without superimposition of the clavicle and may offer valuable clues as to the location and nature of the lesion on the basis of the direction in which it seems to shift on a lordotic film (posterior lesions seem to move downward, anterior lesions upward). Decubitus films allow estimation of the mobility of a mediastinal lesion and may disclose fluid levels not seen otherwise. They may also disclose that the mediastinal widening is due to a mediastinal pleural effusion which shifts away from the center of the chest on decubitus views. Films exposed in inspiration and expiration allow one to appraise the presence and degree of mediastinal shift and the ability of the lungs to expand and contract. Mediastinal abnormalities which produce incomplete bronchial obstruction may produce obstructive emphysema on one side, in which case the affected lung will remain expanded during expiration.

The Valsalva and Müller maneuvers may help the examiner decide that the mediastinal lesion in question is vascular, but these maneuvers are not often helpful.

Other views of the mediastinum may be valuable, and the number of them is limited only by the ingenuity of the physician and technician in placing the patient in such a position that the abnormality will be best displayed. At times, the use of very high kilovoltages will be indicated, and films of the mediastinum exposed with very high kilovolt x-rays generated by a therapy machine may produce highly penetrated films of value in appraising mediastinal abnormalities.

Fluoroscopy is often a sensible procedure to employ prior to the exposure of special films once a mediastinal abnormality is detected on the routine PA and lateral views. By fluoroscopy, one may be able to determine whether or not the lesion pulsates, and if the pulsations are intrinsic (aneurysms, for example) or transmitted (tumor adjacent to the aorta, for example). Moreover, the effects of changes in intrathoracic pressure on the size and shape of mediastinal masses may be directly visualized fluoroscopically, as may the movements of the diaphragm. A mediastinal mass which has interrupted impulses down the phrenic nerve will produce an elevated paralyzed hemidiaphragm on the affected side, a hemidiaphragm which may show paradoxical movement on inspiration.

The relation of mediastinal lesions to adjacent structures may be more easily ascertained at fluoroscopy than on ordinary films, and the swinging of the mediastinum from side to side in patients with a partially obstructed bronchus resulting from a foreign body or tumor may be quite striking at fluoroscopy.

BODY SECTION RADIOGRAPHY

Body section radiography (laminography, tomography and so forth) will seldom disclose the precise nature of the mediastinal mass but may be very valuable in determining its shape and location. Calcifications within the lesion may suggest granulomatous inflammation as the cause, and at times cavities unseen on ordinary films may be uncovered. The relationships of structures to one another and of abnormalities to normal structures may be established with accuracy, and the integrity of the lumen of the tracheobronchial tree may be predicted (Figure 25).

A common diagnostic problem is the determination of the nature of a hilar and adjacent mediastinal mass. Tomography may help in determining the relationship of the lesion to hilar vascular structures, but angiography is certainly better in this regard. A commonly encountered problem is the presence of large hilar vascular structures which are quite normal but which simulate

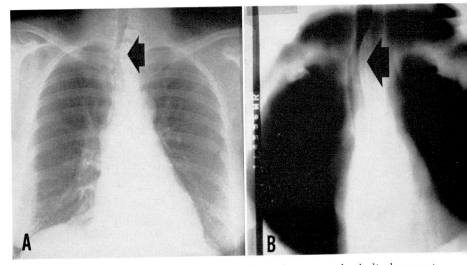

Figure 25. Enlargement of the thyroid producing tracheal displacement. The PA chest film (A) shows localized displacement of the trachea toward the right (arrow) in the region of a mass felt in the neck. Body section radiography (B) shows the displaced trachea and the impression upon it (arrow) more clearly. A nontoxic goiter was found at operation.

hilar lymphadenopathy. Intravenous pulmonary angiography will ordinarily safely and accurately resolve this difficulty.

BARIUM STUDIES OF THE ESOPHAGUS

Except for the study of mediastinal lesions which are clearly located anteriorly and are confined to the anterior mediastinum, opacification of the esophagus with barium is almost always indicated. Intrinsic abnormalities of the esophagus which may produce mediastinal masses or other reflections of mediastinal disease include carcinoma, which usually has characteristic radiologic appearances, and other tumors of the esophagus, including benign tumors if they are sufficiently large. Esophageal leiomyomas and leiomyosarcomas may be sufficiently bulky to displace adjacent structures or bulge laterally in such a way as to deform the mediastinum and be visible on films. Duplication, of the esophagus (enterogenous cysts) rarely communicate with the esophageal lumen, but the barium-filled esophagus may be displaced by a mass which will at least raise the possibility of an enteric or even a neurenteric cyst.

One of the most characteristic appearances of a mediastinal abnormality related to the esophagus is produced by achalasia. Even plain films may display the greatly dilated esophagus projecting to the right of the midline and forming the right mediastinal contour (Figure 26), displacing the trachea anteriorly, and bearing a fluid level in the superior mediastinum. Barium swallow is all that is required to demonstrate the greatly dilated organ, usually containing both fluid and solid particles, and the tapered narrowing at its distal extremity.

More often, barium studies of the esophagus will display reflections of adjacent abnormalities which displace and distort the esophagus. Tumors of all kinds may have that effect, and bronchogenic carcinoma and metastases may in addition invade the esophagus. Lymphomas and neurogenic tumors will more commonly simply displace that organ. Inflammatory mediastinal masses may produce esophageal deformity, and a typical appearance is produced by contracting fibrosing tuberculous mediastinal nodes located at the bifurcation of the trachea which locally retract the esophagus at that level, producing an anteriorly directed traction (and later pulsion) diverticulum. Mediastinitis may produce esophageal distortion and narrowing, as may injuries to the thorax which produce mediastinal hematomas or, later, abscesses.

Vascular abnormalities of the mediastinum are studied with particular profit by opacification of the esophagus, and some mass "lesions" of the mediastinum are shown to be congenital vascular anomalies by study of the barium-opacified esophagus. Right-sided or double aortic arch and anomalies of the subclavian arteries have characteristic esophagographic appearances. Aneurysms displace and deform the esophagus and may offer thereby a clue to their nature.

CONTRAST STUDIES OF THE TRACHEA
AND LARGER BRONCHI

Tracheography and bronchography are not often of great value in the study of mediastinal abnormalities. Intrinsic lesions include carcinoma of the trachea or bronchus which may show a characteristic appearance on opaque studies, and inflammatory masses or strictures may be accurately reflected. Congenital

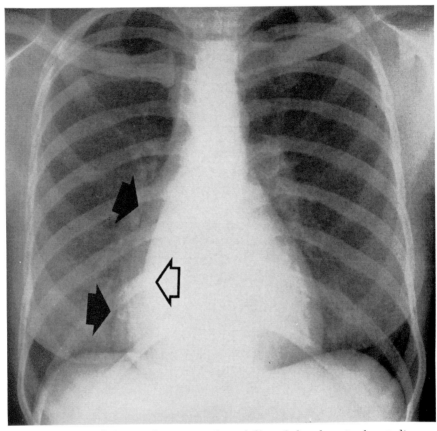

Figure 26. Achalasia. This curious frontal film of the chest is almost diagnostic of achalasia. The hollow arrow points to the right heart border, and the solid arrows point to a mediastinal mass which projects to the right of the heart and which must be located posteriorly since the heart border is not obliterated. The long gentle sweep of the opacity and its medial direction inferiorly are characteristic of the grossly dilated esophagus of achalasia. A barium swallow would make the diagnosis certain.

anomalies of the trachea and bronchi are uncommon but require contrast demonstration for diagnosis.

More often, visualization of the tracheobronchial tree will be valuable for the demonstration of adjacent abnormalities. Aortic aneurysms may displace and deform the trachea or bronchi, and a double or right-sided aortic arch may produce lateral and occasionally posterior compression of the lumen. Anomalous left pulmonary artery (arising from the right pulmonary artery) produces a typical appearance, since it passes between the trachea and esophagus and may be visualized in that location on lateral films. Opaque contrast studies may not be required (naturally occurring air is a good contrast material!). Enlargement of the left atrium may simulate a mediastinal mass, and if the enlargement is sufficiently great, it may widen the angle between the right and left main stem bronchi by elevating the left bronchus, and bronchography may display the abnormality, though plain films are ordinarily sufficient for that purpose.

Other abnormalities may produce tracheal and bronchial distortion such as tumors, particularly lymphomas, bronchogenic carcinomas, metastases to the mediastinum and neurogenic tumors, and contracting inflammatory lesions, often secondary to tuberculous infection. Tension pneumothorax may displace the entire mediastinum, but contrast studies of the airway are unnecessary for its demonstration. Contrast studies may show the presence of a bronchopleural fistula which is located in the mediastinum and which is responsible for the chronic pneumothorax.

PULMONARY ANGIOGRAPHY

Opacification of the pulmonary artery and its branches may be done by either the intravenous or the selective catheter technique, but the intravenous technique has much to recommend it in study of mediastinal abnormalities. Since only the main pulmonary artery and its large major branches are of interest in evaluation of mediastinal disease, the more intense opacification provided by selective studies is unnecessary. Moreover, with the intravenous study one may also examine the mediastinal veins which conduct the contrast agent into the heart.

Intrinsic abnormalities displayed by pulmonary angiography which represent mediastinal disease and which may be profitably studied radiographically include enlargement of the main pulmonary artery and its branches. This may be the consequence of left-to-right shunts which increase the pulmonary vascular volume and produce dilatation of the main pulmonary artery, mitral valve disease, and valvular pulmonary stenosis, with its poststenotic dilatation. It is usually quite obvious that the mediastinal bulge just below the knob of the aorta to the left of the spine represents the dilated pulmonary artery, and angiography is rarely necessary to confirm that impression. Aneurysms of the pulmonary artery or coarctations distal to the pulmonary valve which produce poststenotic dilatation and curious mediastinal shapes may be shown by angiography.

One of the important intrinsic abnormalities of the pulmonary vascular system which requires angiography for accurate display is thromboembolism. At times, this may produce an abnormal opacity on chest films, distorting the mediastinum by virtue of the pulmonary enlargement which may result. In addition, hilar enlargement may be present on one or both sides, the consequence of deposit and buildup of a large volume of clot, producing obstruction peripherally and dilatation proximally and thereby deforming the mediastinum.

Pulmonary angiography is an important diagnostic test in patients suspected of having carcinoma of the lung which is located near the mediastinum. If the vascular contrast study of the pulmonary vessels shows invasion, obstruction or marked distortion of the main right or left pulmonary arteries, the likelihood is great that the lesion is not resectable. Aortic aneurysms may distort the pulmonary artery and its branches and be shown accurately by angiography, and mediastinitis may produce pulmonary vascular obstruction of several types. It may obstruct the pulmonary arteries and thereby mimic carcinoma of the lung, or it may obstruct the pulmonary veins, impede venous return, and result in chronic interstitial pulmonary edema. Vascular contrast studies are required for diagnosis.

AORTOGRAPHY

For the study of mediastinal abnormalities arising from or involving the aorta, intravenous or selective catheter techniques may be used for aortic opacification. The countercurrent method of opacification of the thoracic aorta advocated by some has enjoyed little popularity.

Aortic aneurysms may produce bizarre distortions of the mediastinum, and vascular opacification is required for their accurate diagnosis and for accurate definition of the extent of the lesion. They may be saccular, fusiform or dissecting, and each has its characteristic aortographic appearance. One of the common pitfalls in interpretation of thoracic aortograms in the presence of mediastinal masses results from failure to realize that most aortic aneurysms contain a considerable amount of laminated thrombus on their interior surface, and the opacified lumen is unlikely to correspond exactly with the external shape of the mediastinal mass (see Figure 33). Aortography may also display arteriovenous fistulas arising from the aorta, such as coronary artery fistulas and ruptures of the aorta into cardiac chambers or the pericardium.

Anomalies of the aorta, such as right arch, double aorta and anomalies of origin of the subclavian arteries are best displayed by aortography.

Of all the special procedures available for study of mediastinal abnormalities, probably none is more valuable in planning surgical therapy than aortography, for it defines the lesion as vascular or not in most cases, and if the lesion is not vascular, then the likelihood of discovering its nature short of biopsy is remote.

SELECTIVE ARTERIOGRAPHY

The selective catheterization of vessels within the mediastinum or which supply mediastinal structures for the purpose of injecting contrast material has been performed for some time, particularly bronchial arteriography for the study of lesions of the lung and mediastinum. Thymic tumors and other mediastinal lesions such as teratomas may be studied by selective internal mammary arteriography, and it is likely that the blood supply to lymphomas and other mediastinal masses could be rendered opaque by selective arteriography. To date, this kind of examination has yielded little in the way of practical information, and even bronchial arteriography, once thought to be especially valuable in differentiating neoplastic from inflammatory lesions, leaves a great deal to be desired.

VENOGRAPHY

Since some of the mediastinal contours are normally made up of veins, their opacification may be very valuable in the study of mediastinal abnormalities. Intravenous injections of contrast material which opacify the innominate veins and superior vena cava may show dilatation, displacement or obstruction by adjacent mass lesions such as aneurysms and neoplasms (Figure 27). In

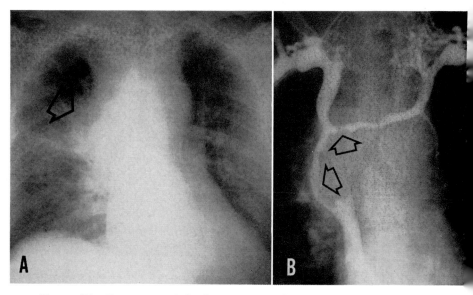

Figure 27. Carcinoma of the lung. Frontal film of the chest (A) shows a large and irregular right hilar and paratracheal mass extending out into the right lung (arrow). Biopsy of a supraclavicular node revealed bronchogenic carcinoma. An intravenous angiocardiogram (B) shows invasion of the left innominate vein (upper arrow) and the superior vena cava (lower arrow) by the malignant neoplasm, indicating that the lesion is almost certainly unresectable.

the case of obstruction, extensive collateral circulation will also be displayed. Venography may also disclose certain anomalies, such as persistence of the left anterior cardinal vein (left superior vena cava) which ordinarily drains into the coronary sinus and may produce an opacity to the left of the mediastinum. Equally important is the use of intravenous contrast injections from the right arm to opacify the right innominate vein in patients with right superior paramediastinal soft tissue masses, particularly old people. These opacities may mimic carcinoma but be due only to a tortuous innominate artery displacing the right innominate vein laterally. An intravenous study which opacifies the innominate vein and includes delayed films which later show the innominate artery opacified will establish the diagnosis of arteriosclerosis with tortuosity rather than neoplasm.

Another important mediastinal vein which may be rendered opaque for diagnostic purposes is the azygos vein. A catheter may be introduced into its orifice from the superior vena cava, or contrast agent may be injected into the marrow cavity of one of the lower ribs (intraosseous venography). Such procedures may disclose mediastinal anomalies, such as azygos continuation of the inferior vena cava (injection into the femoral veins is better for this), and aneurysms of the azygos vein may be displayed. Such aneurysms are rare but may produce mediastinal masses.

The most important indication for opaque azygography is the study of patients with mediastinal neoplasms in order to determine resectability. If the tumor has invaded or obstructed the azygos vein, particularly carcinoma of the lung, then it is probably unresectable.

PNEUMOMEDIASTINUM

Diagnostic pneumomediastinum has been employed to better outline anterior mediastinal masses and to aid in the determination of the location of a lesion (pulmonary or mediastinal). The extent and invasiveness of mediastinal masses or metastases sometimes may be displayed by this technique, particularly when combined with body section radiography. Some employ the study to investigate mediastinal extensions of carcinoma of the lung and to determine the resectability of esophageal carcinoma. Absence of the thymus in immune deficiency states may be shown in this way. But for practical purposes, diagnostic pneumomediastinum is rarely employed, and other studies will usually suffice.

MYELOGRAPHY

Opacification of the spinal subarachnoid space may be necessary to confirm the diagnosis of anterior meningocele producing a mediastinal mass. Neurogenic tumors, arising in the posterior mediastinum, commonly produce distinctive appearances on ordinary chest films, and myelography is rarely required for diagnosis. But when symptoms suggest the neural origin of such a lesion, myelography may be necessary to determine its extent and its effect upon the spinal cord.

PNEUMOPERITONEUM

Introduction of a gas in the peritoneal cavity for diagnostic purposes may at times resolve a diagnostic dilemma. Anterior herniation of bowel or omentum through a patent foramen of Morgagni may be displayed by pneumoperitoneum, thus disclosing the nature of the anterior mediastinal mass seen on routine chest films.

LYMPHANGIOGRAPHY

This procedure has little use in the study of mediastinal abnormalities. At times, the thoracic duct may be visualized, but otherwise it is of little practical assistance.

Chapter 6

THE HEART AND GREAT VESSELS

CONVENTIONAL CHEST FILMS

THE ROUTINE VIEWS of the heart and great vessels include the following: posteroanterior, lateral, and right and left anterior oblique. All of these except the left anterior oblique are commonly obtained with barium in the esophagus. On such films, one can evaluate the size, shape, location and relations of the heart and great vessels, and these four films are usually requested in the initial radiographic study of the patient suspected of having heart disease. Since only a silhouette is seen on ordinary films, only the marginal contours of the heart may be evaluated and the overall shape of the cardiovascular silhouette thereby determined. Much can be learned from such plain films, and at times nothing more is needed in order to confirm a suspected diagnosis or to institute therapy. Indeed, some shapes are so typical as to suggest the correct diagnosis from simple inspection; for example, classical tetralogy of Fallot, large left-to-right shunts, and systemic hypertension (Figures 28, 29 and 30). Such films are also appropriate and valuable for evaluation of the distortion of the heart which may result from abnormalities of the bony thorax, and ordinary films, including the oblique views, are usually all that are necessary to establish the relationship between a mediastinal mass and the heart.

The overall size of the heart may be appraised in a number of ways from conventional films. Most observers simply estimate the size of the heart on the basis of previous experience and describe it as normal, enlarged or borderline. More accurate is use of the cardiothoracic ratio, a figure which assumes that in older children and adults the ratio of the transverse diameter of the heart to the internal diameter of the thorax at the level of the diaphragm will be 50 percent or less. The method is subject to

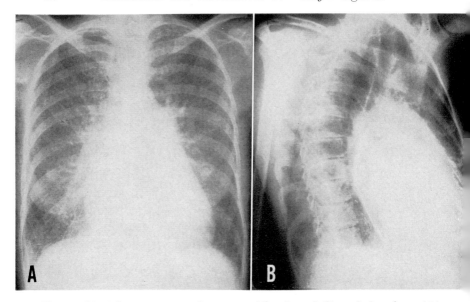

Figure 28. Rheumatic mitral stenosis. The frontal film of the chest (A) shows a prominent main pulmonary artery and a triangular-shaped heart. Shunting of blood into the upper lungs is evident, and costophrenic septal lines, indicating the presence of pulmonary venous hypertension, are seen on the right. The right anterior oblique view (B), made with barium in the esophagus, shows posterior displacement by an enlarged left atrium.

many inaccuracies and is crude at best. More accurate though more tedious is determination of the volume of the heart by applying a formula which includes the length, width and depth of the heart, assuming that organ to be an ellipsoid. Since it considers three dimensions, it gives a more accurate estimation of heart size. Its greatest value also comes from serial determinations used to follow the course of heart disease.

The size and shape of the great vessels in the thorax may also be evaluated in a gross way from plain films. Syphilitic aortic aneurysms are likely to be calcified, and gross enlargements of the pulmonary artery and its branches secondary to obstructive disease on the left side of the heart, left-to-right shunts, and pulmonary hypertension are usually well seen.

The indications for obtaining the routine views of the heart and great vessels are very numerous. The procedure is innocuous

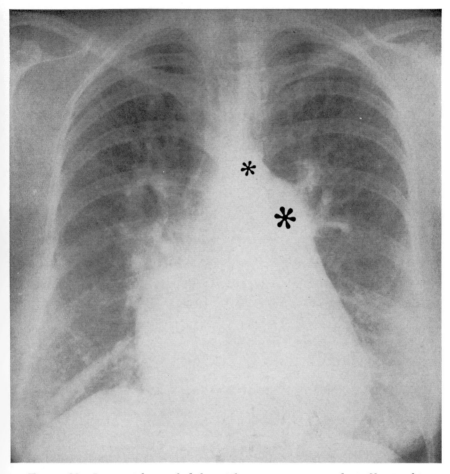

Figure 29. Interatrial septal defect. The posteroanterior chest film in this patient with a murmur since early life shows a small aortic arch (small asterisk) and a very large main pulmonary artery (large asterisk). This is associated with a triangular-shaped heart suggesting right ventricular hypertrophy. In addition, the blood flow to the lungs is increased.

and should rarely be omitted in any patient suspected of having an abnormality of the cardiovascular system.

Special views are occasionally needed. The posteroanterior view of the heart is standard since it minimizes magnification, but if the patient is unable to stand or sit, a recumbent antero-posterior film may be used. This may be especially necessary

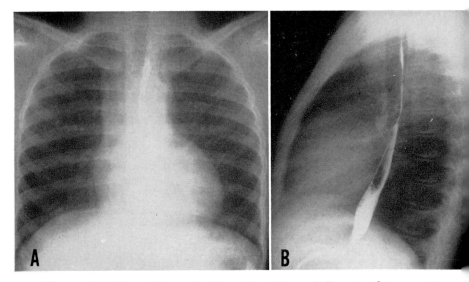

Figure 30. Tricuspid atresia. Frontal and lateral films in this cyanotic young child show no evidence of cardiomegaly but decidedly avascular lung fields. The electrocardiogram showed left axis deviation (unlike what one would find in tetralogy of Fallot). The combination of clinical, radiographic and electrocardiographic evidence strongly points to tricuspid atresia or one of its variants.

when a portable film exposed at the bedside is required because of the patient's inability to come or be transported to the Radiology Department. Specially positioned (sometimes by fluoroscopy) coned-down views of the heart may be indicated at times when the abnormality to be displayed is particularly elusive. A good example is a calcified cardiac valve, demonstration of which requires overexposure of the film, careful positioning, and a very short exposure time.

Under certain circumstances films made in varying degrees of obliquity rather than standard right and left anterior oblique films may prove especially useful. That is particularly true in the evaluation of subtle abnormalities of cardiac shape and size, which are exaggerated in one position only. This may be seen at the time of cardiac fluoroscopy, and appropriate films should be exposed to permanently record the abnormality. Decubitus films may be needed to show fixation of the heart and mediastinal structures or to demonstrate filling and emptying of a pericardial diverticulum or cyst in different positions. The Trendelenburg position is also used in the study of the heart and great vessels, particularly in the evaluation of pericardial effusion. The waist of the heart is said to enlarge with the patient in a head-down position in the presence of pericardial effusion, but that sign is of questionable reliability.

FLUOROSCOPY

Fluoroscopy of the heart and great vessels was once a very popular and much used procedure. As the limitations of the procedure have become better known and as more attention has been paid to the amount of radiation to which the patient is exposed, cardiac fluoroscopy has been performed less; chest films in various positions have largely replaced the procedure. The overall size of the heart and individual chamber enlargement can be better appraised on films of the chest made with barium in the esophagus, and the shape of the heart is probably better appraised that way as well. However, fluoroscopy may be necessary at times for examination of the relations of the heart to adjacent structures, and the fact that the patient may turn from one side to the other during the fluoroscopic examination is an advantage not enjoyed by the use of ordinary films.

Most important is the estimation of the magnitude and character of pulsations of the heart and great vessels. Some experience is required to learn what is normal and that the range of normal is very great.

A hyperactive heart, showing increased pulsations, may be seen in hyperthyroidism, left-to-right shunts, anxiety states, anemia, and at times in pulmonary stenosis. Cardiac pulsations may be diminished in the presence of cardiac failure and pericardial effusion. Regarding the latter, the diagnosis may be established during fluoroscopy if the epicardial fat line can be clearly visualized at some distance deep to the lateral pericardial border. The heart may then be seen to pulsate normally within the fluid which surrounds it. That is an infrequent finding. Cardic pulsations may be diminished over a localized area of the heart where myocardial infarction has occurred. Paradoxical pulsations may at times be seen during cardiac fluoroscopy and are presumptive evidence of ventricular aneurysm.

Two kinds of unusual pulsations of the heart and great vessels have special colloquial designations. "Rocking chair pulsations" are seen in aortic insufficiency; this designation is applied to the exaggerated opposite pulsations demonstrated by the left ventricle and aorta in this condition. "Hilar dance" is applied to the abnormally increased pulsations of the hilar vascular structures in such conditions as atrial septal defect and patent ductus arteriosus.

Fluoroscopy of the heart and great vessels is valuable in the search for cardiac calcifications and is probably the method of choice. Calcifications in the cardiac valves, in the coronary arteries, in the myocardium or pericardium, and in the great vessels may be accurately detected and carefully localized by fluoroscopy.

CINEFLUOROGRAPHY

The recording of the fluoroscopic image of the heart and great vessels on movie film is indicated and valuable when a permanent record of the fluoroscopic findings is desired. It has the advantage that many may study it simultaneously and that it may be compared with previous studies in an objective way. An additional advantage is the ability to play back the movie film at a different rate of speed than it was recorded, slowing down the action when necessary and accelerating it when valuable for visual clarity.

Cinefluorography is specifically indicated for certain abnormalities. These include the search for calcifications in the coronary arteries and heart valves and the demonstration of the epicardial fat line in pericardial effusion.

BODY SECTION RADIOGRAPHY

Because the heart is continuously in motion, body section radiography is unlikely to produce other than a considerably blurred image. Its only important indication in the study of diseases of the heart and great vessels is confirmation of the presence of intracardiac or vascular calcifications, and this is better done by image-amplified fluoroscopy and cinefluorography.

ROENTGEN KYMOGRAPHY

Films may be exposed in such a way that pulsations resulting from several cardiac cycles may be recorded on a film, allowing one to inspect the magnitude and timing of atrial and ventricular pulsations as well as pulsations of the great vessels. This is sometimes employed in an attempt to determine whether or not a mass shows pulsations, and certain characteristic patterns are said to be produced by mitral valve disease and pericardial effusion. For practical purposes the procedure has been abandoned in favor of image-amplified fluoroscopy, cinefluorography and angiography.

CHEST FILMS FOLLOWING INTRODUCTION OF CONTRAST MATERIAL

The exposure of single films of the chest following the introduction of contrast material into the heart or great vessels is rarely indicated and rarely performed. Carbon dioxide angiocardiography may be used with profit in cases of suspected pericardial effusion, and it may be necessary to expose no more than a single film with the patient in the left-side-down decubitus position. This is more usually performed with serial films or with cinefluorography, however. The introduction of opaque contrast material into the heart followed by the exposure of a single film ("single shot" angiocardiography) produces incomplete and often misleading findings. Opaque angiocardiography may be used with profit for pericardial effusion, and while it is true that only a few films need be exposed, a single film may be quite misleading. The same is true for pulmonary angiography in the search for embolism or arteriovenous malformations, for example, and aortography using single film exposures following the injection of contrast material is likely to be inadequate.

Following the removal of fluid from the pericardial sac in cases of pericardial effusion, contrast material, usually air, may be introduced in order to outline the inner surfaces of the pericardium. Under such circumstances the exposure of single films is entirely appropriate and may be quite valuable. PA and lateral films in the erect and decubitus positions as well as the exposure of supine and prone lateral films using a horizontal beam may be quite valuable in demonstrating all of the internal surfaces of the pericardial sac. The indication for such a procedure is the need to determine whether or not the pericardial surface is smooth or is deformed by irregular thickening such as might be seen in pyogenic pericarditis or tuberculosis or with nodules such as might be seen in metastatic malignant neoplasms.

Diagnostic pneumothorax may be induced on rare occasions to search for congenital defects in the pericardium. If present and if the patient is properly positioned, the air used to effect pneumothorax may find its way into the pericardial sac and thereby, by inference, confirm the presence of such a defect.

INTRAVENOUS ANGIOCARDIOGRAPHY

Carbon dioxide angiocardiography is performed in many institutions for the diagnosis of pericardial effusion. The patient is placed with the left side down, and 50 to 150 cc of carbon dioxide are injected intravenously. The gas accumulates in the right atrium and allows estimation of the distance between the inner wall of the right atrium and the outer pericardial density. Thickening in this area suggests pericardial effusion. The method has drawbacks, however, and false negatives are troublesome.

A mixture of carbon dioxide and opaque material is in experimental use for demonstration of the cardiac valves.

Intravenously injected opaque contrast material may be used for the study of diseases of the pericardium, heart and great vessels. Pericardial effusion and thickening (pericarditis) may be demonstrated consistently, when present, by the intravenous injection of contrast agent. The right atrium is opacified, and the distance between the right atrial endocardium and the parietal pericardium may be estimated. Examination is done in the supine position, and a combined thickness of the pericardium and right atrial wall in excess of 4 mm is abnormal (Figure 31).

Angiocardiographic study of heart disease is usually done by the selective technique, the catheter being placed in or near the chamber of interest. However, intravenous angiocardiography, with the contrast material injected into a peripheral vein at a distance from the heart, still has value in certain conditions. It

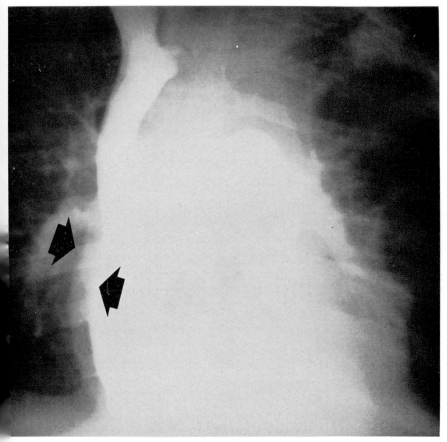

Figure 31. Pericardial effusion (venous anigocardiogram). Contrast material has been injected intravenously, and this film from the serial sequence shows that the inner border of the right atrium (the arrow on the right) is separated from the lateral border of the cardiovascular silhouette (the arrow on the left) by a soft tissue opacity which conforms to the shape of the right side of the heart. A pericardial effusion is responsible for this band of increased density.

may be particularly valuable in very young infants in whom catheterization is hazardous and in others in whom catheterization is difficult or impossible.

Right-to-left shunts in infants are a particular indication for vascular contrast studies, and intravenous angiocardiography may satisfactorily display the altered anatomy in such conditions as tetralogy of Fallot, pseudotruncus arteriosus, transposition of the great vessels, tricuspid atresia and pulmonary atresia. It is emphasized again, however, that when possible, selective studies should be employed.

One of the uses for intravenous angiocardiography is preliminary screening of patients with complex cardiac abnormalities prior to catheterization. Because intravenous angiography is safe and relatively simple to perform, it may be done in advance of cardiac catheterization and selective angiocardiography to guide the examiner during the more definitive study.

Pulmonary valvular stenosis may be studied by the intravenous technique when only gross information is desired. Most often, selective angiography should be employed.

Abnormalities of the great vessels are also ordinarily studied by the injection of contrast material directly into these vessels through a properly placed catheter. However, when catheterization is unusually hazardous or undesirable for whatever reason, intravenous techniques may be successfully employed in carefully selected patients.

Pulmonary thromboembolism may be diagnosed in a number of ways, and in a patient without cardiac failure and with a relatively normal-sized heart, intravenous pulmonary angiography may suffice. Similarly, it may be valuable in pulmonary artery coarctation or in absence or anomalous origin of the pulmonary artery or its branches. In partial or complete anomalous venous return, intravenous angiography may be helpful, as well as in pulmonary arteriovenous fistulas.

Gross abnormalities of the thoracic or abdominal aorta may be adequately demonstrated following the intravenous injection of a large volume of any of the ordinary aqueous iodinated contrast substances. For the demonstration of aortic aneurysms the technique has great value, being simple to perform and quite safe. Intravenous thoracic or abdominal aortography may also be employed for the study of aortic coarctation and for gross obstructions. The intravenous technique should not be used for the study of branches of the aorta, as the degree of opacification is inadequate.

SELECTIVE ANGIOCARDIOGRAPHY

Contrast material is injected through a catheter, the tip of which is placed just proximal to the area of interest. Uniplane or biplane films may be exposed at speeds up to twelve films per second, or cineangiocardiography may be performed at speeds of sixty frames per second or even faster in some recently developed units.

The indications for selective angiocardiography include unusually complex congenital or acquired cardiac abnormalities in which detailed morphological information is necessary or valuable in planning therapy or in venturing a prognosis.

Injections are made into the superior or inferior vena cava if the catheter cannot be advanced into the right atrium or if it is feared that advance of the catheter will dislodge a thrombus or fragments of a tumor. Injections into the right atrium are indicated in Ebstein's anomaly of the tricuspid valve and tricuspid atresia. Contrast material may also be injected into the right atrium when the operator is unable to advance the catheter into the right ventricle for selective right ventriculography.

Right-to-left shunts at the ventricular level and beyond are best studied by selective injection of contrast material into the right ventricle. These include ventricular septal defects and patent ductus arteriosus with reversed flow, transposition of the great vessels, double outlet right ventricle, truncus arteriosus, single ventricle, hypoplasia of the left ventricle and aorta, and tetralogy of Fallot. Obstructive lesions on the right side of the heart also lend themselves particularly well to selective right ventriculography. This includes pulmonary stenosis of all types (Figure 32), including the infundibular pulmonary stenosis seen in Fallot's tetralogy. Selective right ventriculography is also indicated in cases of pulmonary atresia (pseudotruncus arteriosus).

Injections into the right ventricle are required to radiographically demonstrate tricuspid insufficiency, and the rare aneurysms of the right ventricle are also best displayed in this manner. Selective right ventriculography is valuable in postoperative evaluation of patients with congenital or acquired cardiac abnormalities. Right ventricular injections may also be necessary if it is impossible to advance the catheter into the pulmonary artery for pulmonary angiography.

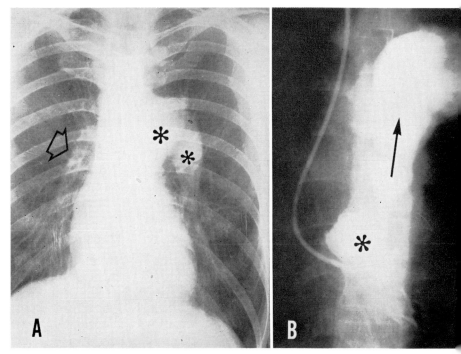

Figure 32. Congenital valvular pulmonary stenosis (ventriculogram). (A) The conventional frontal chest film shows findings which are highly suggestive of pulmonary stenosis. The main pulmonary artery (large asterisk) is enlarged, and its left branch (small asterisk) is similarly enlarged (compare it with the normal descending pulmonary artery on the right to which the arrow points). This combination of large pulmonary trunk and left pulmonary artery with a normal right pulmonary artery strongly suggests the correct diagnosis. (B) A selective right ventriculogram was performed, and the asterisk identifies contrast material in the right ventricle. To either side of the vertical arrow which indicates the direction of flow one can see thickened valve leaflets that do not open adequately during ventricular systole. The great size of the main pulmonary artery is also displayed. Turbulent flow is thought to be responsible for the poststenotic dilatation.

Selective pulmonary arteriography is indicated in patients suspected of having pulmonary thromboembolism and in the study of pulmonary arteriovenous fistulas and anomalous pulmonary venous return, partial or complete. Pulmonary insufficiency may also be judged in this way, and right-to-left shunts through a patent ductus arteriosus or an aortic-pulmonary window may be successfully shown. For valvular pulmonary stenosis, right ventricular injection is indicated. For postvalvular stenosis or co-arctation of the branches of the pulmonary artery, pulmonary angiography is preferred.

Contrast material may be deposited in the left atrium following the introduction of a catheter across the interatrial septum through a patent foramen ovale or by the trans-septal puncture technique. Such injections are indicated in the study of patients with rheumatic mitral stenosis, atrial septal defect with left-to-right shunt, and tumors of the left atrium. At times, it is necessary to inject into the left atrium for the study of abnormalities of the left ventricle and aorta when left ventricular catheterization is impossible, difficult or hazardous.

Selective left ventriculography may be accomplished by injection through a catheter, the tip of which was advanced into the left ventricle across the aortic valve from the aorta, across the mitral valve from the left atrium, or via a needle passed through the chest wall and left ventricular myocardium from the outside. Conditions susceptible to display by left ventriculography and in which the examination may be indicated include mitral insufficiency, endocardial cushion defects, and ventricular septal defects with left-to-right shunt. Obstructions to outflow from the left ventricle are best demonstrated in this way. Such obstructions include idiopathic hypertrophic subaortic stenosis, discrete fibrous subvalvular aortic stenosis, valvular and supravalvular stenosis, and coarctation of the aorta. Left ventricular aneurysms may be shown by this technique, and transposition of the great vessels and tricuspid atresia may be more completely characterized by left ventricular injections.

AORTOGRAPHY AND ARTERIOGRAPHY

The aorta may be opacified intravenously, as previously noted, but most aortography is done by direct injection of the contrast agent into the aorta. Translumbar needle puncture and injection may suffice for the study of aortoiliac occlusive disease, but retrograde catheter aortography (from the upper or lower extremity) is likely to be more thoroughly satisfactory. Catheter study may at times be impossible because of occlusive peripheral vascular disease.

Selective catheter injection of contrast material into the ascending aorta is indicated in the study of aortic insufficiency, valvular and supravalvular aortic stenosis, patent ductus arteriosus, and aortic-pulmonary window. It enables the anatomy of truncus arteriosus to be more thoroughly understood, and it is the examination of choice in the study of coarctation of the thoracic aorta. Aneurysms of the thoracic aorta (Figure 33) and of the proximal parts of the vessels arising from the aorta are also indications for ascending aortography. Arteriosclerotic narrowing of the vessels arising from the arch of the aorta are also demonstrated by this technique, as is "pulseless disease" (Takayasu's arteritis). Dissecting thoracic and abdominal aortic aneurysms may similarly be displayed by selective injection into the aorta.

While midstream injection of contrast agent into the thoracic or abdominal aorta may suffice for the demonstration of branch

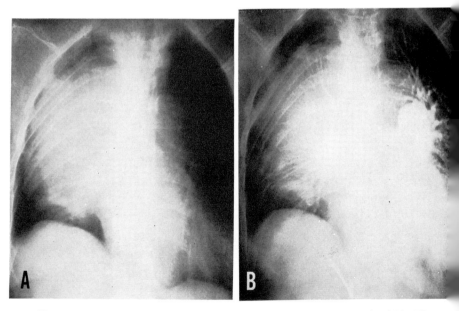

Figure 33 A and B. Aortic aneurysm (venous aortogram). (A) The frontal film of the chest shows a huge mass occupying most of the right hemithorax. (B) Contrast material was injected into the inferior vena cava through a catheter introduced percutaneously into a femoral vein. Its tip can be seen just beneath the right hemidiaphragm. Contrast material in the cardiac chambers shows that the heart has been displaced laterally and inferiorly by the huge mass on the right.

arteries arising therefrom (Figure 34), selective arteriography is more desirable and often indicated. Selective carotid, subclavian and vertebral arteriography may be accomplished by means of special catheters introduced into the thoracic aorta, and the major branches of the abdominal aorta may ordinarily be selectively catheterized with ease. Obstructions, aneurysms, atherosclerosis, injuries and congenital anomalies of these vessels may thereby be displayed. Enlargements and deformities of the abdominal viscera, including tumors and cysts, may be shown by selective arteriography of those vessels. The site of gastrointestinal bleedings may be discovered by selective celiac or superior mesenteric arteriography in a difficult case. Selective bronchial arteriography is of occasional value in the study of mass lesions of the lung.

SELECTIVE CORONARY ARTERIOGRAPHY

Selective coronary arteriography has enjoyed a steadily increasing popularity as a means of accurately mapping the coro-

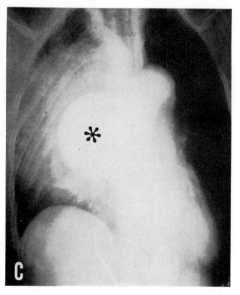

Figure 33 C. A late film from the serial sequence shows contrast material in the thoracic aorta. The asterisk denotes the lumen of the huge ascending aortic aneurysm. The lumen is considerably smaller than the aneurysm, and the remainder of the soft tissue density seen on the frontal chest film is produced by laminated thrombus within the lumen.

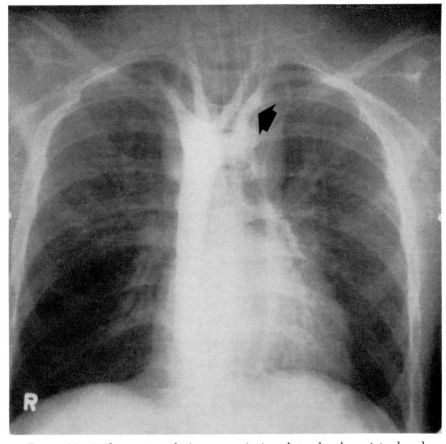

Figure 34. Right aortic arch (aortogram). A catheter has been introduced from below and contrast material injected into the arch of the aorta. The aortic knob is plainly located to the right of the trachea. The arrow points to the aberrant left subclavian artery which arises independently from the right-sided aortic arch. Such an arch commonly produces a posterior impression upon the esophagus, visible by performing a barium swallow.

nary circulation. It is indicated in the study of patients with unusual chest pain in whom coronary artery disease is a distinct possibility but the diagnosis is uncertain. It is an important adjunct in patients with angina pectoris and a normal or unusual electrocardiogram, and it is an essential part of the process of patient selection for surgical treatment to relieve the symptoms of coronary insufficiency. One of its most important applications is the demonstration of a normal coronary artery circulation in patients previously thought to have arteriosclerotic heart disease on the basis of history, symptoms or suggestive electrocardiographic findings. In such patients the cause for chest pain can be sought elsewhere, and the patient can be reassured that coronary artery disease severe enough to produce angina is not present. The catheter may be introduced through the brachial artery by cutdown or by the percutaneous transfemoral approach. Either is satisfactory and, in experienced hands, successful in a very high percentage of cases (Figure 35).

PERIPHERAL ARTERIOGRAPHY

Peripheral arteriography of the extremities by needle puncture or catheterization is indicated chiefly for the study of ischemic peripheral vascular disease, ordinarily on an arteriosclerotic basis. The character and extent of obstructive disease may be elegantly demonstrated, along with the collateral vessels by which flow is redirected distally. Arteriography of the extremities is also of importance in the study of injuries to blood vessels and in the late effects of these injuries, such as arteriovenous fistulas. Tumors of bone and soft tissue arising in the extremities may be studied arteriographically with profit, their nature and extent thereby being disclosed.

VENOGRAPHY AND VENACAVOGRAPHY

Peripheral venography is indicated in the study of the anatomical consequences of thrombophlebitis and prior to surgical or other therapy for varicose veins. Displacement and obstruction of veins resulting from tumors and injuries may also be shown by venography of the extremities and of the pelvis. Tumors of the mediastinum, particularly carcinoma of the lung, may obstruct the superior vena cava, and contrast material injected into upper extremity veins on each side will disclose the location and extent of the obstruction as well as the collateral flow around it.

Abdominal masses may produce vena caval displacement, distortion or obstruction, and venacavography may be valuable in their preoperative evaluation. Thrombi within the pelvic veins or

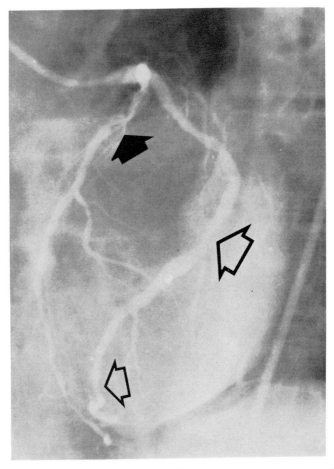

Figure 35. Coronary arteriogram (selective coronary arteriogram). The branches of this dominant left coronary artery show numerous areas of irregular narrowing (hollow arrows), particularly in the larger circumflex artery. The anterior descending artery is very narrow and irregular, particularly proximally (solid arrow).

inferior vena cava as a source of emboli to the lung may also be displayed (Figure 36).

At times, it will be necessary to selectively catheterize the renal veins in cases of suspected renal vein thrombosis, but there is a minimal hazard in this procedure, as the clots may be dislodged.

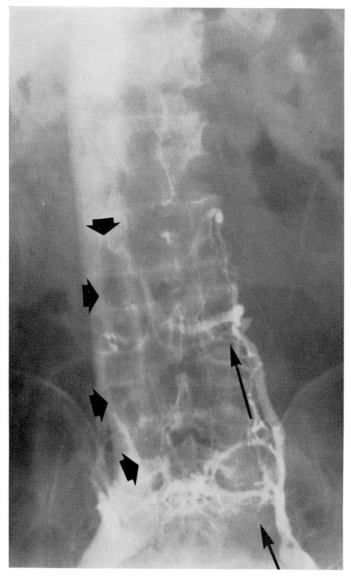

Figure 36. Thrombosis of the inferior vena cava. Contrast material was injected into both femoral veins simultaneously. The contrast material injected into the patient's right femoral vein outlines an elongated radiolucent filling defect within the inferior vena cava which is a large thrombus (small arrows). The contrast agent injected on the left entered the ascending lumbar veins (long arrows), eventually joining the inferior vena cava above the area of thrombosis.

Chapter 7

THE GASTROINTESTINAL TRACT

ORDINARY (PLAIN) FILMS OF THE ABDOMEN

ONE USUALLY THINKS of barium studies of the gastrointestinal tract as the definitive examinations for the detection of diseases and abnormalities, but it is wise to begin the radiographic examination of the intestinal tube with plain films. Certain abnormalities are susceptible to diagnosis by plain films alone, and on some occasions information obtained by examination of the ordinary films will contraindicate certain kinds of contrast studies (oral administration of barium in high-grade colon obstructions, for example).

Recumbent anteroposterior and erect films of the abdomen are the first studies usually ordered. On such films the gastrointestinal gas pattern may be inspected, and the soft tissue shadows of the spleen, liver and kidneys may often be discerned and are a key to their size, shape and location. The lateral margins of the psoas muscles may be examined, and the fat layer superficial to the peritoneum permits us to indirectly inspect this serous membrane in the flanks. Opaque calculi and abnormal calcifications may be detected. Displacement of intra-abdominal organs by abnormal masses may also be discovered.

For several reasons the recumbent film is almost always more valuable than the erect film. First of all, it is easier to obtain, requiring less patient cooperation. Secondly, it may be impossible to see both the entire diaphragm and the entire pelvis on a single erect film in many adults. When that is the case, it is the diaphragm that likely will not be shown, and thereby one of the values of the erect film will be lost. Finally, the erect film is more subject to misinterpretation than the recumbent film, particularly in the matter of fluid levels in the bowel. Though much has been written to the contrary, many persons still believe that air-fluid levels on an erect film of the abdomen signify intestinal obstruction. That is certainly not the case; such fluid levels may be found in adynamic ileus, gastroenteritis, following enemas, and in other conditions. Thus, the ordinary supine anteroposterior film of the abdomen, sometimes called a KUB film, will be much more valuable for the preliminary inspection of the intestinal tract, and if one had to choose a combination of films with which to begin, one would select the KUB film of the abdomen and an erect film of the chest (to show air free in the peritoneal cavity collected beneath the diaphragm).

Some of the more common gastrointestinal abnormalities which may be displayed on ordinary films of the abdomen include the following:

1. Paralytic or adynamic ileus, generalized or segmental.

Irregularly arranged, moderately dilated gas and fluid-filled bowel loops are seen in generalized adynamic ileus, and the entire bowel is involved. Bowel loops often overlap one another in this condition, unlike the classical appearance in mechanical intestinal obstruction. In segmental ileus, localized loss of bowel tone occurs, with distention secondary to localized inflammatory disease complicated by neighborhood peritonitis. This produces the appearance of a "sentinel loop," a single, moderately dilated loop of bowel, usually in the midabdomen, commonly the consequence of pancreatitis or cholecystitis. Another kind of nonobstructive dilatation of bowel which can be appreciated on ordinary abdominal films is vascular occlusive ileus, with distention of the small bowel and colon as far as the splenic flexure. One may also see nodular marginal soft tissue encroachments upon the lumen resulting from hemorrhage into the wall of the bowel in this condition which may follow thrombosis of the superior mesenteric artery or some of its branches. Similar changes may occur in the descending colon and sigmoid when the inferior mesenteric artery is affected.

2. Mechanical intestinal obstruction.

The cardinal radiographic sign of mechanical intestinal obstruction on plain films of the abdomen is abnormal and often marked distention of bowel loops, ordinarily selective distention of those loops proximal to the obstruction with little or no air distal to that point. The obstructed bowel loops commonly assume an orderly, disciplined arrangement, often resembling a stack of coins or a stepladder, in contrast to the lack of organization seen in bowel dilatation associated with adynamic ileus (Figure 37). Some of the causes of mechanical intestinal obstruction have specific and diagnostic appearances on plain films of the abdomen. In volvulus of the sigmoid, for example, plain films will often show a greatly distended loop of colon in the shape of an inverted U rising up out of the pelvis and filling much of the abdomen. In volvulus of the cecum a greatly distended cecum may be found just beneath the *left* hemidiaphragm.

Certain congenital anomalies of the intestine producing mechanical obstruction in the newborn period have characteristic radiographic appearances on plain films. Duodenal atresia (with or without annular pancreas) should be suspected when the stomach and duodenal bulb are severely distended and no gas is found distal to the duodenum (the "double bubble" sign). Contrast studies are usually unnecessary to make this diagnosis, though it may sometimes be necessary to aspirate fluid contents from the stomach with a soft rubber catheter and introduce a small amount of air before the abdominal films are made. In ileal atresia in the newborn, dilated intestinal loops will be found to the level of the obstructed bowel. Meconium ileus produces intestinal obstruction when the abnormal gummy and viscid meconium fails to pass normally through the bowel, and if perforation occurs, meconium peritonitis ensues. Calcification of the meconium-soiled peritoneum may produce the diagnostic combination of bowel obstruction and extraluminal calcium deposits in the newborn which makes the diagnosis certain.

Proper use and interpretation of the plain films of the abdomen in small infants with congenital anomalies producing mechanical intestinal obstruction will often obviate the need for other diagnostic studies and permit surgical therapy to be undertaken without delay. There is little of value to be gained by performing a GI series in an infant with typical radiographic features of duodenal atresia on plain films of the abdomen. The delay necessitated by the additional examination merely allows

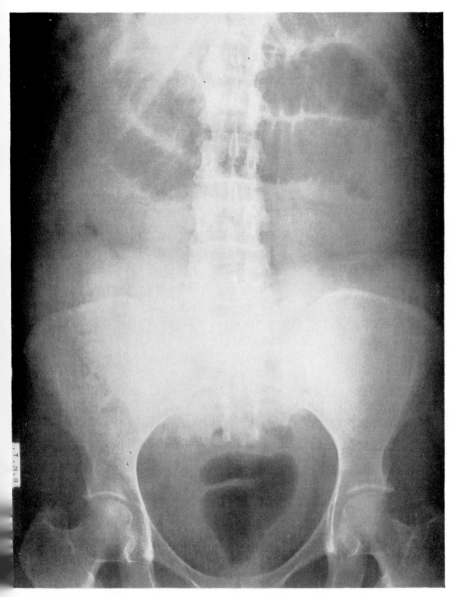

Figure 37. Intestinal obstruction. Greatly dilated loops of small bowel are seen in the upper abdomen, and very little gas is seen distal to that point (the gas in the rectum may have been introduced at the time of digital examination). The dilated small bowel loops have assumed an orderly arrangement sometimes compared with a stack of coins, and the loops do not overlap. At operation a mechanical small intestinal obstruction due to adhesions was found.

time for further dehydration and electrolyte imbalance to occur.

The bowel may be obstructed by foreign materials, such as ingesta, worms and gallstones. The diagnosis of ascariasis may be suspected from the appearance of numerous arcuate radiolucencies representing gas surrounding collections of worms in the intestine. A characteristic roentgen picture is produced when a gallstone erodes its way into the duodenum and finally obstructs the distal ileum. On an ordinary film of the abdomen, dilated small intestine is seen, and if the calculus is opaque, it may be visible in the right lower quadrant. Air (from the bowel) in the biliary tree solidifies the diagnosis.

3. Calculi.

Stones may be found in the gallbladder, biliary ducts, pancreas, appendix, and small and large intestine and in the genitourinary tract. Most stones in the biliary tract are nonopaque; most in the urinary tract are opaque. Calcifications within the pancreas usually signify chronic relapsing pancreatitis. An appendicolith may occasionally offer a clue as to the etiology of obscure abdominal pain.

4. Free air.

The ordinary or plain film of the abdomen is the examination usually chosen for the detection of free air in the peritoneal cavity. While massive amounts of air can be detected on the recumbent film, a film made with the x-ray beam horizontal is usually required. Probably the best film for this purpose is an erect chest film. It will always include the diaphragm and show the collection of free air beneath it (Figure 38). An erect film of the abdomen is commonly requested under these circumstances, and it may be quite satisfactory too. However, because of the difficulty of positioning with the patient erect, particularly if he is very sick, the diaphragmatic dome may not be included.

If the patient is unable to stand, then one of a number of other views may be obtained which will show free air in the peritoneal cavity. The simplest of these (for the patient) is an across-the-table lateral film made with the patient lying supine. Free air will accumulate beneath the peritoneum anteriorly and superiorly and may be seen separately from gas within the bowel. A usually more satisfactory study is the right or left side down

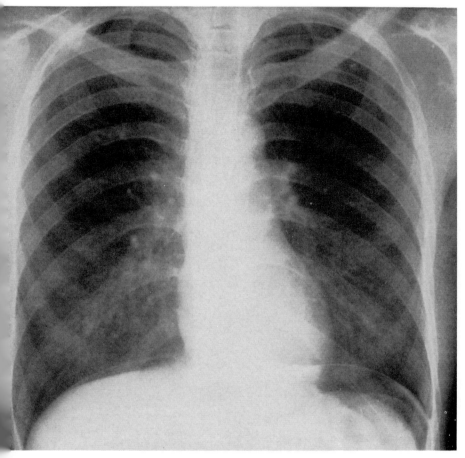

Figure 38. Free peritoneal air. The upper aspect of each hemidiaphragm is outlined by air in the lungs, and in this patient the inferior aspects are outlined by air free in the peritoneal cavity. The most common cause of spontaneous pneumoperitoneum in an adult is perforated duodenal ulcer. An erect chest film is the most satisfactory and reliable way of demonstrating this finding.

decubitus film. The patient lies on either side, and the horizontal x-ray beam passes through the patient from front to back (or from back to front). Free air collects beneath the peritoneum and outside the bowel and is seen in one or the other flank on such a film.

The most common cause of spontaneous pneumoperitoneum

in an adult is perforated duodenal ulcer; in a newborn infant, rupture of the stomach is a more common cause. The appropriate film studies for detection of evidence of a perforated hollow viscus have been outlined above. It is not reasonable to administer barium by mouth under such circumstances. The barium may find its way into the peritoneal cavity, and while barium is not more irritating to the peritoneum than gastric secretions and food, the presence of barium in the peritoneal cavity may make the surgeon's job a good deal more difficult should an operation be required.

GI SERIES

The GI series is the basic x-ray study in the investigation of most symptoms of gastrointestinal origin. A liquid barium sulfate-water mixture is administered by mouth, and its passage through the proximal intestinal tract is monitored by fluoroscopy and spot films or cinefluorography, followed by several films made at the conclusion of the examination. The esophagus, stomach and duodenum are examined with care. The following are some of the more common abnormalities susceptible to display by a GI series:

1. *In the esophagus.*

Ulcerations (commonly resulting from reflux esophagitis in the presence of hiatus hernia); neoplasms, usually malignant, usually carcinoma (Figure 39); strictures, usually a consequence of lye ingestion; displacements resulting from extraesophageal mediastinal masses such as aneurysms and neoplasms; pharyngeal and esophageal diverticula (congenital weakness of the wall, traction resulting from fibrosis in adjacent lymph nodes, and so forth); and uncommon diseases, such as achalasia and scleroderma.

2. *In the stomach.*

Hiatus hernia; benign peptic ulceration; neoplasms, usually malignant, usually carcinoma (Figure 40); polyps; displacements resulting from extragastric masses, particularly tumors or cysts in the pancreas but also pathological enlargement of the liver, spleen and left kidney; unusual tumors, such as leiomyomas and leiomyosarcomas; other unusual lesions such as aberrant pancreas and bezoars; and postoperative changes and complications (gastroenterostomy, marginal ulceration, fistulas).

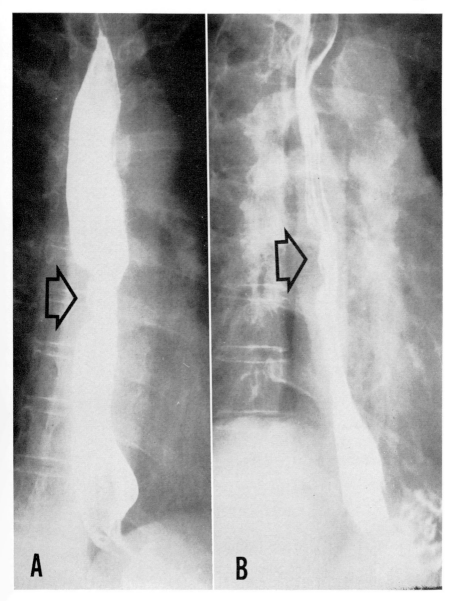

Figure 39. Carcinoma of the esophagus (G.I. series). The arrow points to a localized sessile lesion arising from the wall of the midportion of the esophagus and surmounted by a central ulceration (arrows). The frame in A shows the distended esophagus, and B shows the appearance after the bolus of barium has passed. Observe that the lesion is sharply localized and that the esophagus is normal above and below it.

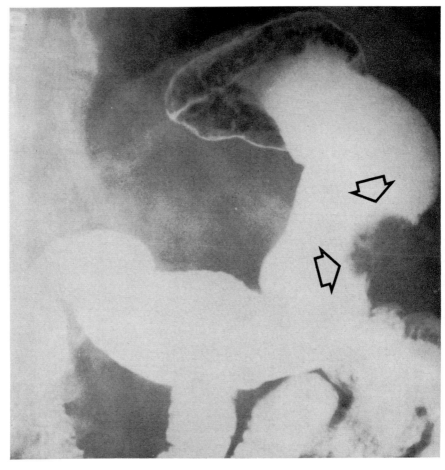

Figure 40. Carcinoma of the stomach (G.I. series). Arrows point to a sessile, fungating radiolucent mass which projects into the lumen from the greater curvature of the stomach.

3. *In the duodenum.*

By far the most common lesion is the duodenal ulcer, usually found in the bulb or in the immediate postbulbar area (Figure 41). Spasm and mucosal edema resulting from duodenitis without ulceration may be found. Diverticula are common and usually trivial. Polyps are uncommon, and malignant neoplasms are very rare. Carcinoma of the ampulla of Vater may project into the

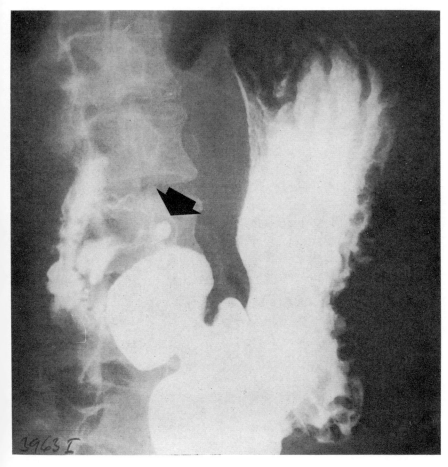

Figure 41. Duodenal ulcer (G.I. series). The stomach is normal in appearance, but the duodenal bulb is markedly deformed. The arrow points to barium within a duodenal ulcer crater. Mucosal edema adjacent to the ulcer niche has nearly filled the duodenal bulb, accounting for the lack of much barium within it.

duodenal lumen as a filling defect, and tumors and cysts of the common bile duct, pancreatic head, gallbladder, liver, right kidney, and other retroperitoneal structures may displace and deform the duodenum, as many aneurysms of the abdominal aorta and intramural hematomas following trauma or in patients being treated with anticoagulants.

The indications for a GI series are very liberal, and the study should be done if the patient's symptoms are thought possibly to arise from the upper GI tract. As a screening test in asymptomatic persons, it is of dubious value.

Follow-up examinations of the GI tract are important in a number of circumstances. The healing of a gastric ulcer should be carefully followed radiographically, for if it fails to heal, an ulcerated carcinoma may be responsible for the radiographic deformity and the patient's symptoms rather than a benign peptic ulcer. Most physicians will want to follow the healing progress of duodenal ulcers by repeat upper gastrointestinal examinations as well. It may be reasonable to omit follow-up examinations in a patient known to have chronic duodenal ulcer disease in whom a classical active ulcer crater has been demonstrated radiographically and who is responding with rapid relief of symptoms to appropriate therapy.

Another important indication for follow-up examination of the GI tract is the failure to find an abnormality in the face of continued symptoms and continued suspicion on the part of the referring physician that a structural abnormality is responsible. Hiatus hernias and esophageal varices may be radiographically visible on one occasion and not on another, and an active duodenal ulcer crater may have been obscured by a tiny blood clot at the first study but plainly seen on a follow-up study. If symptoms and strong suspicion of an abnormality persist after a negative upper GI series, the examination should probably be repeated.

SMALL BOWEL SERIES

This examination is usually accomplished by following the ingested barium sulfate solution during its passage through the intestinal tract by serial large size (14 by 17 inches) films, ordinarily at hourly intervals, with fluoroscopy employed whenever inspection of the films suggests the need for it. Mouth-to-colon transit time is ordinarily about three to four hours, but in some normal patients it may be as short as thirty minutes or as long as seven or eight hours. By virtue of the characteristic appearance of the mucosal surface of the jejunum and of the ileum, lesions found can usually be fairly accurately localized.

Examples of abnormalities susceptible to detection by the small bowel series include the following: polyps, benign and malignant neoplasms, intussusception, malrotation, submucosal malignant infiltration resulting from lymphoma, tuberculosis, regional enteritis, periappendiceal abscess (distorts and displaces the terminal ileum and cecum), Meckel's diverticulum, displacement or invasion by adjacent masses (abscesses, neoplasms), and other rarer abnormalities.

In general, the small bowel series is less productive of valuable information than the GI series and is commonly ordered only after the GI series and barium enema have failed to disclose the source of the patient's symptoms.

BARIUM ENEMA

After careful preparation to obtain a clean colon, a barium sulfate-water mixture is introduced from below, and the colon is filled in a retrograde manner under fluoroscopic control. Spill into the terminal ileum or appendix is desirable in order to be certain that the colon has been completely filled. Preevacuation and postevacuation films are exposed, and spot films or cinefluorograms may be made during the examination to insure that all parts of the bowel have been carefully examined.

Examples of abnormalities which are satisfactorily displayed on such examination include the following: carcinoma (Figure 42), diverticulosis and peridiverticulitis, benign strictures and stenoses, chronic nonspecific ulcerative colitis and ulcerative colitis resulting from tuberculosis and amebiasis, Hirschprung's disease and other varieties of megacolon, polyps, intussusception, volvulus (plain films will ordinarily suffice for the diagnosis), metastases, and lesions of other organs which deform the colon from without (for example, tumors of the ovary, uterus, liver).

The air-barium double contrast enema is a special kind of enema in which the colon is coated with barium while its lumen is distended with air. Such an examination displays small polyps better than the ordinary barium enema, but the air-barium double contrast enema is probably not the examination of choice for other abnormalities, and its reputation among some as a "deluxe" barium enema is probably undeserved. A good examination requires that the colon be meticulously clean.

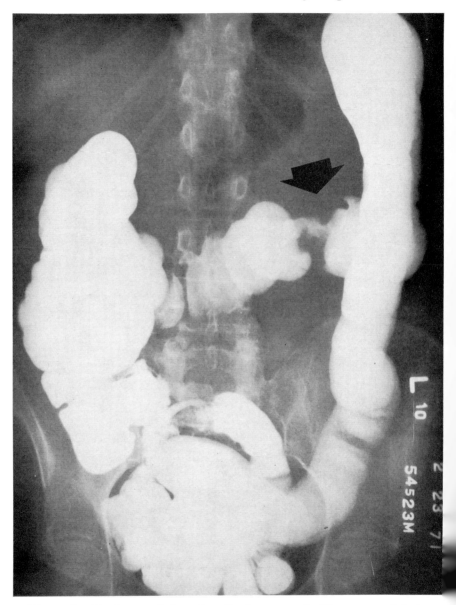

Figure 42. Carcinoma of the colon (barium enema). The arrow points to a lesion in the transverse colon characterized by a rigid constricted lumen. The lesion begins and ends abruptly, and overhanging edges are seen on both extremities of this sharply localized and absolutely typical-looking annular adenocarcinoma.

Specific indications for barium enema include changes in bowel habits and rectal bleeding. Anemia, pain and unexplained diarrhea are common indications as is weight loss and a mass in the abdomen. Suspicion of colon disease is sufficient indication, but it is probably not worthwhile to order the examination only for "completeness" of the GI workup.

At times, the barium enema examination may be employed for therapy, deliberately or inadvertently. Hydrostatic reduction of intussusception is an accepted mode of therapy and probably the most gentle way to reduce an intussusception. Infants with the meconium plug syndrome may be relieved of their symptoms and caused to expel the obstructing plug by the stimulus of a barium enema.

ORAL CHOLECYSTOGRAM

The usual x-ray examination of the gallbladder is begun by the administration of special contrast material by mouth the night before. Time is allowed to elapse while the contrast agent is absorbed from the intestine, excreted by the liver, and concentrated in the gallbladder (usually overnight). The following morning films are exposed of the right upper quadrant. A normally functioning gallbladder becomes intensely opaque under these circumstances, and calculi within the lumen may be easily discerned. Indeed, stones are about the only serious abnormality of the gallbladder displayed by oral cholecystography, though on occasion cholesterol polyps, myoepithelial anomalies and very rarely carcinomas may be seen. Most gallstones are nonopaque, and they are not displayed on ordinary films of the abdomen but instead are seen as radiolucent filling defects within the contrast-filled gallbladder (Figure 43). When cholelithiasis is strongly suspected but the gallbladder functions poorly, it may be sensible to administer the ordinary dose of contrast substance daily for a few days. Under such circumstances some of the contrast material is adsorbed onto the surface of the stones, rendering them visible on films of the abdomen.

In the presence of chronic cholecystitis, the capacity of the gallbladder wall to absorb water and therefore to concentrate the opaque material may be so impaired that the gallbladder is

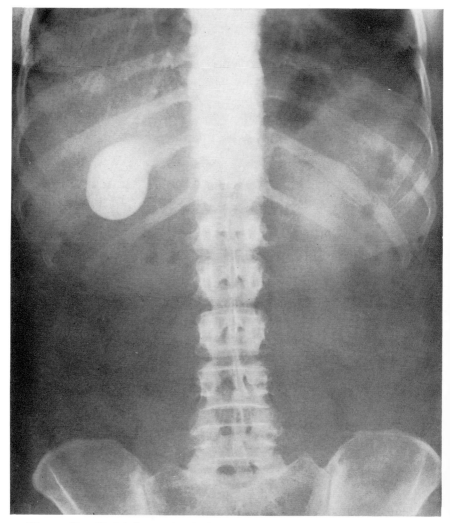

Figure 43. Cholelithiasis (oral cholecystogram). The frontal film of the abdomen shows numerous facetted radiolucent stones within the opacified gallbladder. Most gallstones are not radiopaque and require cholecystography for their demonstration.

not visualized by oral cholecystography. A more common cause of nonvisualization of the gallbladder is failure of the patient to take the tablets the night before. Other causes must also be taken into consideration. The patient may take one or two tablets, vomit them, and take no more. Or the patient may take all of the tablets and then ingest his usual nightly laxative, which may speed the passage of contrast material through the intestine so rapidly that not enough is absorbed to opacify the gallbladder. Juxtapyloric obstruction may cause the contrast material to remain in the stomach (duodenal ulcer is a common cause), or hepatocellular disease may prevent the excretion of contrast material sufficiently rapidly or in high enough concentration to be seen. In the presence of a moderately to markedly elevated serum bilirubin, one does not expect the gallbladder to be visualized by oral cholecystography, and some other form of examination may be attempted.

Because oral cholecystography requires at least several hours to perform, it is uncommonly employed in the evaluation of a patient with acute abdominal symptoms requiring urgent therapy. It is indicated in the diagnostic workup of a patient with symptoms thought to be due to gallbladder disease. Gallstones and nonvisualization are by far the most common abnormalities detected. The diagnostic accuracy of oral cholecystography, when positive, is among the highest of any radiographic study.

OTHER GALLBLADDER AND BILIARY TRACT EXAMINATIONS

When the gallbladder has been surgically removed and visualization of the biliary system is desired, *intravenous cholangiography* may be performed. This examination may also be done when the gallbladder is present if reliable information regarding gallbladder function and structure is desired within a relatively short period of time (about two hours). In a patient with severe right upper quadrant pain, visualization of a normal-appearing gallbladder by intravenous cholecystocholangiography largely excludes cholecystitis as the cause (since this is most often associated with an obstructing calculus in the cystic duct). The intravenous route of administration of contrast material may also be employed when the oral route is unavailable or unsatisfactory for any reason (pyloric obstruction, diarrhea, persistent vomiting, gastrocolic fistula, for example).

In the presence of high-grade obstructive jaundice or severe hepatocellular disease, neither oral nor intravenous examination are likely to be of value. In such cases *percutaneous transhepatic cholangiography* may be attempted. Under local anesthesia a needle is inserted into the liver percutaneously and then slowly withdrawn until bile can be aspirated through it. As much bile as possible is removed, and contrast material is injected directly into the biliary ducts. The patient is then positioned appropriately, and several films are exposed. These will most often show a dilated duct system and the cause of the obstruction, usually a stone (Figure 44) or neoplasm in the common duct, a stricture, or a tumor in the head of the pancreas. If repeated attempts fail to permit aspiration of bile, one may conclude with fair reliability that the biliary duct system is not dilated and that the jaundice is on a hepatocellular basis (hepatitis, for example).

Percutaneous transhepatic cholangiography should be performed only after consultation with the surgeon. Should obstructive jaundice be found, the patient should be operated upon promptly and the biliary system decompressed by whatever surgical procedure is indicated. Otherwise, bile peritonitis is likely to ensue from leakage of bile around the needle because of the high pressure in the biliary duct system. For that reason it is also wise to leave the needle used for cholangiography in the duct system for temporary decompression while the patient is being readied for operation. A flexible needle-catheter (such as a Teflon® or Rochester needle) is ideal for such a purpose.

SELECTIVE VISCERAL ARTERIOGRAPHY

Modern techniques permit relatively easy selective catheterization of the celiac, superior and inferior mesenteric arteries, followed by injection of contrast material and serial filming. Such studies may be extremely valuable in the problem case and may display a variety of abnormalities. Selective celiac arteriography is especially valuable for the study of neoplasms of the liver, primary and metastatic. Hepatomas show a characteristic vascular tumor stain or blush, and metastatic nodules may be either vascular, as in the case of disseminated carcinoid, or avascular and show only displacement of vessels, as in metastases from carcinoma of the pancreas. Pancreatic tumors may be diagnosed with

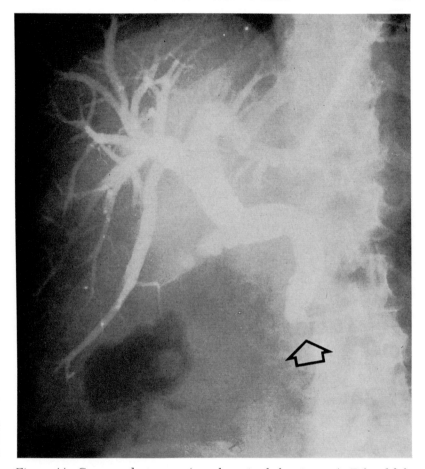

Figure 44. Common duct stone (transhepatic cholangiogram). Dilated bile ducts are opacified by contrast material introduced through a needle placed percutaneously into the liver. The arrow points to the complete obstruction produced by a radiolucent gallstone in the distal end of the common duct. A superiorly convex meniscus defines the proximal edge of the stone, and all of the biliary radicals proximal to that are dilated.

confidence from a selective celiac arteriogram when the tumor has affected the vessels which course within and adjacent to the pancreas (displacement, obstruction, tumor encasement, tumor vessels, and tumor stain). In a jaundiced patient with a negative or equivocal GI series, the choice between selective celiac arteriography and percutaneous transhepatic cholangiography must be made. Valuable information may be obtained with either procedure, but it must be remembered that transhepatic cholangiography requires immediate surgical exploration if positive. Nevertheless, one is more likely to obtain information of value by cholangiography than by arteriography.

Selective celiac arteriography may also be employed in the search for occult bleeding sites in the bowel, particularly in the stomach and duodenum, and superior mesenteric arteriography may be used for the same purpose in the small intestine and proximal colon. Barium studies of the intestine are usually employed first, but if they are negative and the patient continues to bleed, selective visceral arteriography should be seriously considered. The patient must be actively bleeding at the time the study is performed, or it is likely to be negative.

For the study of abdominal angina or vascular occlusive ileus, abdominal aortography is preferred, with filming in the lateral projection so that the origins of the celiac and superior mesenteric arteries may be seen. High-grade stenosis of the superior mesenteric artery near its origin plus similar stenosis of either the celiac or inferior mesenteric arteries are necessary before abdominal symptoms may be attributed to vascular insufficiency. The collateral circulation between the three large visceral arterial trunks is so extensive that stenosis or obstruction of only one of them is unlikely to result in symptoms.

Abdominal aortography may also be used to establish the diagnosis of aneurysm. The intravenous technique may be used, but in most patients the retrograde catheter technique may be used safely and is preferred. Translumbar aortography is probably also satisfactory, but one runs the risk of puncturing the aneurysm with the needle, and the examination provides a great deal less versatility for positioning than the other methods. Aortic aneurysms may produce GI symptoms and signs by pressure or by erosion or rupture into the lumen of the bowel.

Selective visceral arteriography is of value in the patient who has suffered blunt trauma to the abdomen if the nature and extent of the injury are in doubt. Splenic and hepatic rupture, lacerations, and subcapsular hematomas may be accurately demonstrated.

SPLENOPORTOGRAPHY

This study consists of percutaneous puncture of the spleen followed by the injection of contrast material and serial filming over the abdomen to display the venous drainage of the spleen and the portal venous circulation. Its use is largely limited to the study of patients suspected of having portal hypertension, usually resulting from hepatic cirrhosis. In a normal patient the contrast agent flows directly from the splenic pulp through a non-dilated splenic vein into the portal vein and thence into the intra-hepatic portal radicles. In portal hypertension the splenic vein is likely to be dilated, and collateral venous channels bypass the liver. These circuitous collaterals may take many courses, and a common finding is reflux of contrast material from the splenic vein up the coronary veins and thence into gastric and esopha-geal varices. Numerous other pathways are possible (Figure 45).

Bleeding from the spleen into the peritoneal cavity is a rare

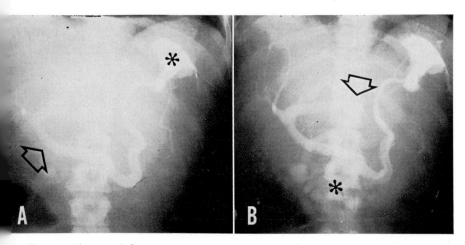

Figure 45. Portal hypertension (percutaneous splenoportogram). (A) A needle was introduced percutaneously into the splenic pulp where contrast material was deposited (asterisk). The contrast agent is immediately taken up by the splenic vein which drains into the portal vein (arrow). (B) A slightly later frame in the serial sequence shows retrograde filling of the recanalized umbilical vein via a much enlarged left branch of the portal venous system (arrow). The asterisk marks the serpiginous dilated um-bilical vein which forms a caput medusae which may be visible on the skin surface.

but possible complication following the examination, and the study should not be performed unless surgical consultation has been obtained and the possibility of splenectomy considered. While we always take this precaution, we have yet to encounter a case in which bleeding from the spleen following precutaneous splenoportography has required emergency surgery.

The portal venous system may be opacified in other ways, but they are much less commonly employed. Hemorrhoidal veins may be directly injected, and films will then display the superior mesenteric or inferior mesenteric venous systems and then the portal vein. Contrast material may be injected directly into the superior mesenteric venous tributaries during operation. In some patients the umbilical vein may be surgically exposed, dilated and catheterized, and contrast material may be directly deposited into the left portal vein or even into the main portal vein if the catheter can be advanced far enough.

The splenic and portal venous systems may also be opacified by superselective celiac arteriography. The catheter is advanced through the celiac artery and into the splenic artery, where contrast material is selectively deposited. Delayed filming will show the splenic parenchyma, splenic vein and portal vein.

One other use to which splenoportography has been put is the study of suspected tumors of the body and tail of the pancreas which may be visible on the basis of their effect upon the splenic vein which runs just superior to this part of the pancreas. Neoplasms and pancreatitis have been known to produce irregularities, displacements and obstruction of the splenic vein in this vicinity.

OTHER VENOGRAPHY

Rarely is inferior venacavography required in the diagnosis of diseases and abnormalities of the GI tract. Occasionally, opacification of the vena cava may be valuable in displaying the relationships of an abdominal mass and its effect upon venous return. Occasionally, direct hepatic venography may be attempted by passing a catheter from an arm vein down the superior vena cava, and then directly into the hepatic veins. Contrast material deposited here satisfactorily outlines in a retrograde manner the hepatic venous system and may show effects of mass lesions within the liver to good advantage. On occasion, it may also display thrombosis of one or more hepatic veins (Budd-Chiari syndrome). Wedged and free hepatic vein pressures may also be determined by this technique, allowing an estimation of sinusoidal pressures to be made. These figures may be of value in making decisions about the need for and type of operative treatment in patients with portal hypertension.

DIAGNOSTIC PNEUMOPERITONEUM

Though rarely employed and rarely indicated, the introduction of gas into the peritoneal cavity may occasionally be of value in the diagnosis of diseases of the gastrointestinal tract. A right upper quadrant opacity may be an enlarged liver or a normal-sized liver and a subpulmonic effusion. Defining the location of the diaphragm with peritoneal gas may resolve the difficulty. Intramural mass lesion of the fundus of the stomach may elude definition by ordinary GI series but may be plainly seen when surrounded with gas in the peritoneal cavity. The size and shape of the spleen may be accurately displayed by diagnostic pneumoperitoneum, though it should rarely be necessary. In general, the examination is reserved for complex diagnostic problems in which simpler studies have failed to adequately demonstrate the size, shape, location or nature of a suspected abnormality so that therapy may be undertaken.

Several gases have been employed. Carbon dioxide is rapidly absorbed and readily available.

PANCREATOGRAPHY

Of all of the organs of the GI tract, the pancreas remains the most elusive. Reference has already been made to the usual means of examination (GI series, celiac arteriography, splenoportography), but no method is entirely satisfactory since no technique has yet been devised to render the organ homogeneously and safely opaque. Retrograde injection into the pancreatic duct after catheterization of the ampulla of Vater is gaining in popularity as a means of diagnosis. Efforts to increase and then opacify the secretions of the pancreas have been insufficiently successful to permit clinical application. The combination of retroperitoneal gas insufflation and diagnostic pneumoperitoneum (sometimes additionally with celiac arteriography or barium studies of the intestinal tract) still leave much to be desired and at best allow the impression of enlargement or irregularity of the pancreas. In practice, the pancreas is examined indirectly by means of the usual upper gastrointestinal series or at times by means of hypotonic duodenography. In this latter procedure the duodenal loop is temporarily paralyzed with a potent para-sympatholytic drug, and films are exposed of the duodenum distended with air and coated with barium. Lesions of the head of the pancreas may thereby be better displayed. If after these studies disease of the pancreas is still imperfectly displayed, celiac arteriography and transhepatic cholangiography may be attempted.

Chapter 8

THE URINARY TRACT

RECUMBENT ANTEROPOSTERIOR FILM
OF THE ABDOMEN (KUB)

THE BASIC FILM STUDY of the urinary tract is the supine frontal film designed to show the soft tissues in the abdomen, particularly the kidneys, ureters and bladder (KUB).

The KUB film serves many purposes and should not be omitted as the preliminary roentgenologic study of the urinary tract regardless of what procedures follow. Renal size and shape may be appraised, largely because of the perinephric fat which surrounds and defines the outer margins of the kidneys. Displacement of the kidneys and (occasionally) distortions of their shape may be seen. Of great importance is the ability to visualize opaque calculi within the urinary tract (Figure 46), and on carefully positioned, well-exposed films in which the exposure time is short and movement is minimized, one should expect to see even tiny calculi located within the renal parenchyma (nephrocalcinosis), the collecting structures of the kidneys (nephrolithiasis), the ureters, and the bladder. About three fourths of the calculi in the urinary tract are opaque to roentgen rays; the KUB film, therefore, becomes one of the most valuable film studies for their detection.

The margins of the iliopsoas muscles are often sharply defined by adjacent retroperitoneal fat. Asymmetry in these shadows and particularly marginal irregularities or localized absence of the density of the psoas margin may be an important indicator of retroperitoneal disease. Tumors and abscesses in particular may invade the retroperitoneal fat about the psoas muscles and obliterate their margins radiographically. Calcifications along the course of the psoas muscles seen in association with destructive disease of the spine are characteristic of tuberculous spondylitis with abscesses.

113

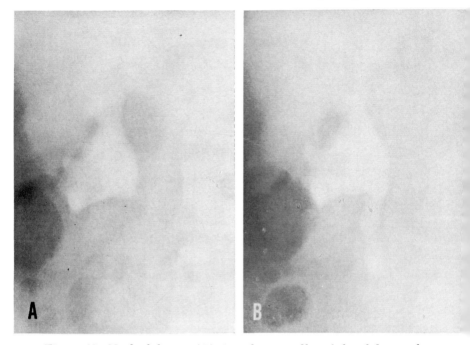

Figure 46. Nephrolithiasis. (A) A preliminary film of the abdomen shows the presence of a staghorn calculus within the right kidney collecting system. Most renal stones are opaque, as is this one. (B) Following the intravenous injection of contrast material one can observe that some function remains in the right kidney for the contrast material has been excreted and can be seen in the right ureter. It is also obvious that the staghorn stone nearly completely fills the collecting system on the right.

Certain neoplasms associated with the urinary tract produce characteristic calcifications which may be easily visible. Chief among these are carcinomas of the kidney, 15 to 20 percent of which contain radiographically visible calcium. These malignant tumors are more likely to contain calcium than are benign renal cysts (less than 5%). Neuroblastoma of the adrenal is also characteristically associated with filmy and irregular calcifications, and this tumor may produce downward displacement of the kidney if the neoplasm is sufficiently large. Wilm's tumor of the kidney may contain calcium from time to time, but its most characteristic appearance on a plain film of the abdomen is displacement of gas-filled bowel loops to the opposite side by what is ordinarily a sizable mass. The psoas shadow on the involved side may also be obliterated or deformed.

Other abnormal calcifications associated with the urinary tract may be seen on a simple frontal film of the abdomen. Calcifications in atherosclerotic aortic plaques may be found in patients with stenotic lesions of the orifices of visceral arteries, including the renal arteries. Renal artery aneurysms often contain calcium in their walls which assumes the configuration of an incomplete circle and is seen near the renal hilus. Arteriovenous malformations or fistulas within the kidney may also be calcified and visible on plain films. Calcified phleboliths in the pelvis rarely are confused with stones in the urinary tract because of their characteristic tiny radiolucent center. Stones seen below the line between the ischial spines are almost always phleboliths if not located in the midline. Exceptions are stones in the urinary bladder or prostate, but their appearance and location ordinarily leave no doubt as to their identity.

By virtue of its contrasting density with adjacent structures, gas in the urinary tract may be plainly visible. Urinary tract infections with gas-forming organisms, particularly in diabetic patients, may produce gross amounts of gas within the lumen of the bladder, within the wall of the bladder (cystitis emphysematosa), in the ureters and in the kidney collecting systems. Such amounts of gas commonly produce rather subtle radiologic findings, but at times, the volume of gas in the renal pelvis may be so great as to permit confusion of its appearance with bowel gas, and consequently, the lesions may be overlooked. A more dramatic diagnostic appearance is cast by perinephric abscesses when sizable amounts of gas are formed within them. The gas takes the form of numerous small bubbles which do not coalesce and which do not change their position relative to one another as the patient changes position. Because of this they produce an appearance unlike that of gas in the bowel, and when a sizeable collection of these tiny bubbles is seen in the region of the kidney, particularly when the margins of the kidney are invisible or indistinct, one should suspect the presence of perinephric abscess.

EXCRETORY UROGRAPHY (IVP)

Excretory urography is the simplest contrast examination of the urinary tract and is in itself usually adequate for diagnostic purposes. The patient is prepared for the examination by administration of a laxative the night before or enemas the morning of the study and by withholding the meal preceding the examination. Fluids are ordinarily allowed in usual amounts until shortly before the examination, and it is probably unnecessary and potentially harmful to dehydrate the patient prior to urography. Particularly in patients with marginal renal function, dehydration is likely to be detrimental, and it may precipitate overt renal failure in patients with multiple myeloma. The enhanced contrast which may result from dehydration is frequently balanced by incomplete opacification of the urinary tract because of the small urine volume, and most examiners now prefer to use a larger volume of contrast material in a normally hydrated patient.

The examination should not be left entirely in the hands of the technician following the injection of contrast material. A physician should remain in the vicinity to treat reactions even though they are infrequent. He should also be present to judge the need for additional views or for prolongation of the procedure past twenty minutes when indicated. Oblique views will be important on occasion to separate the opacified renal collecting systems from overlying opacities, gallstones, for example. Oblique or even lateral views may also be valuable in determining the size and shape of masses which deform the collecting systems. When excretion is slow, as in the case of obstructive uropathy, delayed films may be necessary to display adequately the anatomy of the collecting structures and the nature of the obstructing lesion. This delay may be as long as twenty-four hours in certain circumstances. In some patients, particularly in children, where it may be routine, the administration of a carbonated beverage by mouth will distend the stomach with gas and permit enhanced visualization of the collecting structures of the kidney. Some examiners, finding poor opacification of the collecting structures with an ordinary dose of contrast material, will make a second injection of the contrast agent during the conduct of the study. Prone and decubitus films may occasionally be indicated, and the decision to modify the routine must be left in the hands of the radiologist.

Excretory urography is indicated in patients having no contraindication to the procedure in whom there is suspicion of disease of the urinary tract. This suspicion will most often be raised by complaints such as frequent or painful urination, cloudy or dark colored urine, the passage of stones or "gravel," suprapubic pain or tenderness or a feeling of fullness, pain in the back or flank, and hesitancy in starting the stream or diminished force of urination. Other symptoms suggest systemic manifestations of renal disease such as azotemia, edema, hypertension, or symptoms of infection which might originate in the urinary tract. Signs of urinary tract diseases which indicate the need for excretory urography include hematuria, pyuria, abdominal masses (particularly in children), and objective signs of infection, hypertension or renal decompensation. Abnormalities disclosed by analysis of the urine in the asymptomatic individual also call for radiologic study. Excretory urography is also indicated in many special circumstances, as in the search for a primary site of malignant disease in the presence of distant metastases, following injury to the abdomen or back, in the workup of candidates and donors for renal transplantation, and others. Indeed, there are few instances in which suspicion of disease or abnormality of the genitourinary tract should not be pursued by excretory urography.

The contraindications are few. The only absolute contraindication is unusual sensitivity to the contrast material, and the examination should not be performed if the patient has previously experienced a severe reaction to iodine. A careful history of responses to the ingestion or injection of iodine-containing materials should always be obtained, and a small intravenous test dose is commonly used. However, a negative response to the intravenous injection of 1 ml of contrast material one to two minutes prior to the remainder of the dose is no guarantee of safety, and a test dose followed by one or two skin wheals or by nausea may not indicate hypersensitivity or necessitate discontinuing the procedure. A relative contraindication is renal failure with an elevated blood urea nitrogen of such a level that satisfactory visualization of the renal collecting structures cannot be anticipated (BUN more than 80 mg per 100 ml). However, it is often surprising how satisfactory a study can be obtained with delayed films even in the face of a moderately elevated BUN. Rather than using average or smaller than average doses in the presence of renal failure, larger doses of contrast material are often necessary once it has been decided that excretory urography is an important study to undertake in the individual patient. There is no evidence that the intravenous injection of large doses of contrast substances is dangerous in these patients. Although excretory urography is a relatively safe procedure, it is not recommended as a screening test or as a part of the work-up of the patient who presents himself for an annual or other "checkup." A relative contraindication, then, is the lack of a valid indication for the procedure.

The kinds of abnormalities susceptible to demonstration by excretory urography are as follows:

INTRINSIC DEFORMITY OF COLLECTING STRUCTURES. Congenital anomalies may result in deformities of the collecting structures which present such distinctive radiographic patterns as to allow specific diagnosis by excretory urography. These include horseshoe kidney, crossed ectopy, bifid collecting systems, pelvic kidney (Figure 47), and congenital hypoplasia. Infection results early in ureteral dilatation and calyceal enlargement and later in marginal irregularities, strictures and stenoses, and permanent calyceal deformities and dilatation. One of the characteristic manifestations of chronic pyelonephritis demonstrated by excretory urography is the scarred and pitted cortex which is greatly diminished in thickness in areas of severe infection and atrophy. Certain infections may produce characteristic radiologic appearances (such as tuberculosis), but for the most part individual organisms do not produce sufficiently characteristic changes to permit their specific identification. Infection of the urinary bladder must ordinarily be quite severe to produce changes on excretory urography. In such cases nodular mucosal edema and hyperplasia may be visible as marginal smooth or irregular filling defects in the contrast-filled bladder. Neoplasms produce some

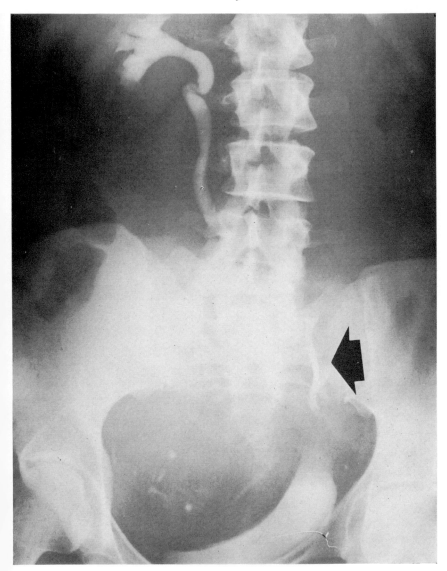

Figure 47. Pelvic kidney (excretory urogram). The arrow points to the opacified pelvis and calyces of an ectopically located kidney on the left. The right kidney collecting system is normal except for being minimally dilated. The cause is obvious from inspection of the impression upon the dome of the urinary bladder produced by an early and unsuspected pregnancy (some of the fetal bones can be seen).

of the most striking and severe intrinsic deformities of the collecting structures or other portions of the urinary tract. Kidney cysts may displace and deform adjacent collecting structures and produce rounded nodular swellings on the cortical surface. Malignant neoplasms invade and destroy the renal parenchyma, producing both displacement and deformity from destruction of parenchymal tissue and the associated collecting structures. Malignant neoplasms of the ureter have an appearance not unlike that produced by carcinoma of the bowel and are usually localized lesions, sometimes showing overhanging edges. Tumors of the bladder produce filling defects within the opacified lumen, but this is often better shown by retrograde cystography than by excretory urography.

EXTRINSIC DEFORMITY OF COLLECTING STRUCTURES. Renal cysts ordinarily produce changes in the excretory urogram by compressing and distorting the collecting structures from without. Such cysts are ordinarily rounded, are often multiple, may be bilateral, and may cause the outer cortex of the kidney to bulge. The opacified collecting structures are ordinarily displaced and draped over and around the cysts rather than being invaded and destroyed as with a malignant neoplasm. Cysts or tumors of adjacent organs may also produce extrinsic deformities of the collecting structures, and adrenal masses are especially likely to depress the kidney on the affected side. Other retroperitoneal masses may have a similar effect. An enlarged spleen commonly produces mild extrinsic deformity of the left kidney; if the enlargement is massive, it may actually displace the left kidney from its normal position. Masses in the pelvis and lower retroperitoneal area may cause displacement of the ureters, and infraperitoneal tumors and masses may dislodge the bladder from its usual position.

FILLING DEFECTS. *Neoplasms,* in addition to their tendency to displace and distort adjacent collecting structures, may invade the lumen of the kidney pelvis, infundibula, or calyces and may thereby be visualized as a negative or radiolucent filling defect within the opacified lumen. Such tumors may appear as a similar filling defect within the ureter, some polypoid and some sessile. Filling defects in the bladder from neoplasms are uncommonly

pedunculated and are usually represented on the excretory urogram by a diffuse and irregular thickening of a localized portion
of the inner surface of the bladder. *Stones* may be found in any
part of the kidney collecting system and are usually opaque and
visible on the preliminary film. They appear as filling defects
within the contrast-filled renal collecting and storage structures,
and unless opaque stones are more dense radiographically than
the contrast material, they may appear relatively radiolucent
within the contrast-filled lumen, despite the fact that they are
opaque on the KUB film. Stones which remain for any length
of time in the urinary bladder are commonly faceted because
of abrasion with adjacent stones. The only other common filling defect to be found in the urinary tract is clotted *blood*. Such
radiolucent defects resulting from blood clots are uncommonly
encountered anywhere but in the upper urinary tract. Perhaps
that is because they are evacuated from the bladder with
more or less dispatch. It may occasionally be impossible to distinguish between neoplasm, radiolucent stone, and blood clot by
excretory urography. Very much less common filling defects to
be found from time to time in the urinary bladder are foreign
bodies, and a great variety of bizarre materials has been seen at
one time or another in the bladder, including such things as
paper clips, catheter and catheter pieces, hair pins, pieces of
razor blades, and chewing gum. Another filling defect which is
occasionally seen in the bladder and which has a characteristic
radiologic appearance on excretory urography is ureterocele. It
is a herniation of the distal end of the ureter into the bladder,
ordinarily associated with a stenotic orifice. It appears as an
opaque filling defect with a radiolucent ring surrounding it and
may vary from a few millimeters in size to many centimeters.

OBSTRUCTION. Excretory urography is the method of choice
for the radiologic demonstration of obstructions, though some
will require more sophisticated studies for complete description.
Congenital or developmental abnormalities may produce obstruction by valves, flaps, bands and diaphragms in the urethra or in
the ureters and by distortions in renal architecture which may
make drainage from the collecting structures difficult or impossible. In this category one includes ureteropelvic junction obstruc-

tion resulting from extrinsic bands or from accessory or anomalous vessels which cross in this region and produce incomplete obstruction to drainage from the kidney. Infection may produce urinary tract obstruction obvious on excretory urography by swelling of the mucosa near orifices (as at the ureterovesical junction) or by inflammatory strictures. Stones may obstruct completely or incompletely, and a characteristic sign on excretory urography may allow the diagnosis of acute obstruction of the ureterovesical junction by a calculus, even if the calculus is invisible. Following the injection of contrast material the uninvolved side becomes promptly opaque. Excretion of contrast material is markedly delayed on the involved side, and a dense nephrogram may appear, indicating acute and marked elevation of pressure within the collecting structures, preventing the entrance of contrast material from the renal tubules in the parenchyma into the calyces and pelvis. Neoplasms may obstruct the urinary tract but more often produce their radiologic effects by invasion, distortion and destruction. Extrinsic lesions may produce urinary tract obstruction with some frequency, particularly masses in the pelvis unrelated to the urinary tract which may produce obstruction by involvement of the ureters. A prime example is carcinoma of the cervix which, when widespread in the pelvis, may eventuate in urinary tract obstruction and uremia.

DRIP-INFUSION PYELOGRAPHY

A modification of excretory urography which offers the prospect of denser opacification and more complete filling of the urinary tract than ordinary urography depends upon the infusion of a large volume of contrast material. One milliliter of contrast substance per pound of body weight is mixed in an equal volume of normal saline or 5% glucose in water. It is infused in eight to ten minutes. Films are exposed three and seven minutes following the start of the infusion and then at the conclusion of the infusion and five minutes later at which time an erect postvoiding film can be made if desired. The specific film sequence and timing should be modified according to the indications and findings, however, and no rigid schedule is advised.

Preparation does not differ from that employed for ordinary

excretory urography. The examination as described is more expensive than the usual study because of the large volume of contrast material employed, and it is not suggested that this examination be used routinely. It is indicated when more detailed information is needed regarding the kidney collecting apparatus following less than absolutely satisfactory conventional excretion urography. The sizable volume of fluid employed insures an adequate urinary output and good distention of the collecting structures. The large volume of contrast material assures good opacification. While 1 ml of contrast material per pound of body weight is employed as a rule, under no conditions is more than 150 ml used.

Drip-infusion pyelography, because of the ordinarily superior degree of opacification and contrast filling of the collecting structures, has in large measure obviated the necessity for retrograde pyelography in cases where ordinary excretory urography fails to demonstrate with sufficient clarity the nature of an abnormality. The technique has much to recommend it by comparison with retrograde pyelography: there is a low incidence of untoward reactions, only a venipuncture is necessary rather than catheter manipulation in the ureters, the possibility of infection or reflex urinary shutdown is avoided, and the necessity for general anesthesia is eliminated. It is emphasized that certain diagnostic problems will remain largely insoluble unless retrograde pyelography is employed, but in most instances the drip-infusion technique will be adequate.

NEPHROTOMOGRAPHY

Nephrotomography is the word used to designate body section radiography of the kidneys. It is a technique which deliberately blurs radiographic images outside of the selected plane of interest (that plane being parallel to the table top). This is accomplished by connecting the roentgen ray tube with the Bucky tray containing the film cassette by means of a rigid bar, the fulcrum of which can be varied at will. The roentgen ray tube and film move during the roentgen ray exposure (which lasts several seconds), and their movement in opposite directions around a preselected level of rotation accomplishes blurring of the image above and below the plane of interest. By appropriate settings this plane of interest may be 0.1 to 1.0 cm thick, ordinarily quite adequate for diagnostic purposes.

The usual plane of the kidneys is located 5 to 8 cm from the posterior body wall. Because the kidneys are inclined at a slight angle to the long axis of the body, their upper poles being more dorsal, several "cuts" at close intervals may be necessary to display the entire renal architecture on each side.

Nephrotomography is indicated when greater detail of the retroperitoneal soft tissues is sought. Since it accentuates the contrast between soft tissues and surrounding fat, it is particularly useful in the study of abnormalities of renal shape or in searching for retroperitoneal tumors, particularly of the adrenal gland. Since it blurs the overlying images of gas and feces in the bowel, nephrotomography may be valuable in producing clearer delineation of structural abnormalities present in the collecting systems, and the combination of intravenous urography or drip-infusion pyelography and nephrotomography is a particularly fruitful one. In many cases drip-infusion pyelography combined with body-section radiography of the kidneys will be all that is necessary to establish the diagnosis of solitary or multiple benign renal cysts; in such cases the renal parenchyma will appear opaque, and the cysts will appear as sharply defined, rounded radiolucencies (Figure 48). The appearance of tiny calcifications within the kidney may also be enhanced by this technique.

RAPID SEQUENCE INTRAVENOUS PYELOGRAM AND THE PYELOGRAM-UREA WASHOUT TEST

The excretory urogram may be modified to provide a valuable screening test for suspected renovascular hypertension. Following the intravenous injection of contrast material (50 ml of 50% or 75% Hypaque®), films are exposed at thirty seconds and one, two, three, five, eight and fifteen minutes. If the eight-minute film shows the development of a satisfactory pyelogram on both sides, a fifteen-minute film is exposed as a baseline, following which a solution containing 40 gm of urea in 500 ml of normal saline (for an adult) is infused over a fifteen-minute period, during and following which films are exposed at the rate of one

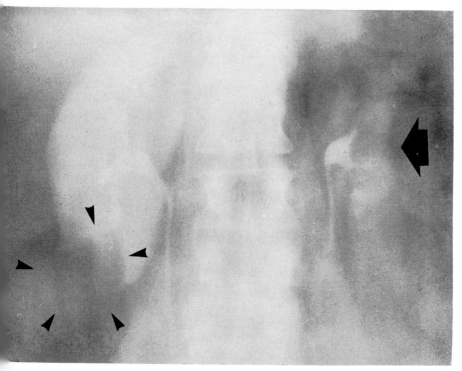

Figure 48. Benign renal cyst (nephrotomogram). Body section radiography has been performed following the intravenous injection of contrast material. The collecting structures on the right are normal in appearance, but the arrowheads point to a rounded radiolucency representing a benign avascular lower pole cyst on the right. The large arrow on the left points to a deep pitted scar due to atrophic pyelonephritis. The rounded calcification above the arrow on the reader's right was due to a splenic artery aneurysm. All of these findings are better displayed on this nephrotomogram than they were on conventional abdominal films.

every three minutes. This filming continues until eighteen to twenty-one minutes following the start of the urea infusion. Immediately following the procedure the patient is rehydrated orally and intravenously, and the examination is concluded.

The film exposed thirty seconds after the start of the contrast injection normally shows good nephrograms bilaterally, that is, it will show contrast material within the renal capillaries and tubules prior to being excreted into the calyces and pelvis, giving the renal parenchyma an overall increased density on each side. From such a film one can determine renal size and shape as well as compare the lengths of the kidneys. The subsequent films exposed at one-minute intervals allow comparison to be made between the two sides regarding the rapidity of excretion. The later films prior to the urea infusion allow the examiner to inspect the morphology of the kidney collecting systems. The early films may well be limited to the kidneys with attention to shielding of the gonads, but the preliminary film and the film exposed at fifteen minutes should be full-sized 14- by 17-inch films.

Infusion of urea provokes an intense and immediate osmotic diuresis. In the normal patient this results in prompt and symmetrical dilution of the contrast material in both kidney collecting systems with prompt "washout" of the pyelogram on each side. Since the usual aqueous iodinated contrast materials employed for urography are filtered by the glomeruli and not reabsorbed by the tubules, increased urine volume produces contrast dilution and the appearance of a rapid washout.

In the patient with a main renal artery stenosis (for example) as the cause of systemic hypertension, the thirty-second film may show a disparity in renal size, the affected kidney being smaller. The early minute-sequence films may show more prompt excretion of the contrast agent on the normal side than on the smaller affected side. The characteristic physiologic abnormality in renovascular hypertension is the rapid reabsorption of water (and sodium) by the affected kidney. The films exposed in such a patient following the start of urea infusion will show prompt dilution of the contrast material and washout of the pyelogram on the normal side as a consequence of the increased urine flow. However, on the affected side the rapid reabsorption of water will maintain the density of the contrast material (since it is not also reabsorbed), despite the osmotic diuresis. A positive washout test, therefore, shows retention of the contrast material in the collecting system on the affected side with prompt washout on the opposite normal side.

The minute-sequence pyelogram and the pyelogram urea washout test are modifications of the standard excretory urogram. They are valuable in screening patients suspected of having renovascular hypertension prior to renal arteriography. The washout portion of the test is, in a sense a radiographic split renal function test (Howard test). Provided that appropriate measures are taken to rehydrate the patient following the examination, complications and untoward reactions are negligible. The patient occasionally experiences chilliness and headache during the urea infusion, but this seldom requires therapy or cessation of the test.

RETROGRADE PYELOGRAPHY AND CYSTOGRAPHY

Following the introduction of catheters into the urinary bladder through a cystoscope, their tips may then be introduced into the ureteral orifices on each side and a catheter advanced into each ureter. Alternatively, cone-tipped catheters may be used to obturate the ureteral orifices in the bladder. In either case, following the retrograde introduction of contrast material, films subsequently obtained can be depended upon to produce superior delineation of detail of the renal collecting structures, including the ureters. A preliminary or scout film is always obtained, and this is followed by films exposed after varying degrees of filling of the collecting structures, in varying obliquities as necessary, following the withdrawal of the catheters and after voiding. Such a sequence of films will demonstrate the flexibility and distensibility of the collecting apparatus as well as its capacity for rapid and complete drainage.

Retrograde pyelography is indicated when the simpler and more benign methods of examination of the urinary tract, involving for the most part the intravenous injection of contrast material, fail to portray adequately the morphology of the kidney collecting structures. It will seldom be necessary to resort to retrograde pyelography if drip-infusion pyelography and nephrotomography are employed. However, there will be occasions when the brilliant contrast and superior clarity available and regularly obtained by retrograde pyelography are essential to proper diagnosis (Figure 49). For example, if one kidney fails to excrete the contrast material entirely in a patient being studied for hypertension and the retrograde pyelogram shows a nor-

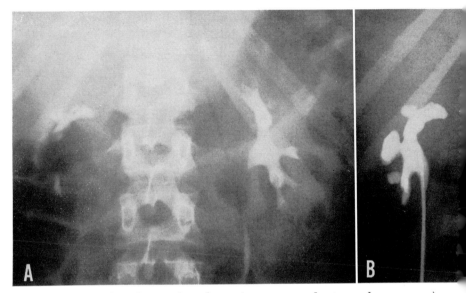

Figure 49. Atrophic pyelonephritis (excretory and retrograde urograms). (A) Excretory urography shows a normal collecting system on the left side. The right kidney is much smaller than normal and shows blunted and deformed calyces, but visualization is incomplete. (B) Retrograde pyelography on the right defines with greatly improved contrast and definition the blunted and deformed calyces in this small, atrophic chronically infected kidney.

mal kidney collecting system on that side, then renal artery stenosis of high-grade or complete obstruction is very likely. Another indication for retrograde pyelography is hypersensitivity to the intravenous injection of iodine-containing contrast substances. When visualization of the collecting structures of the urinary tract is nonetheless important, one may resort to retrograde pyelography.

There are certain hazards and risks in retrograde catheterization of the ureters and bladder. The test is uncomfortable for the patient unless general anesthesia is employed, in which case the admittedly minor risks of that procedure must be considered. Retrograde infection of the urinary tract and the possibility of reflex urinary shutdown must also be considered. For the latter reason some examiners prefer to perform retrograde pyelography on only one side at one sitting, though that is not a universal practice. In skillful hands and in patients with appropriate indications, retrograde pyelography will provide information obtainable by no other means and is an important part of the diagnostic armamentarium in the study of diseases of the urinary tract.

The bladder is regularly visualized following the intravenous injection of contrast materials, but intravenous cystography is unlikely to be regularly of great value. The bladder is not often distended by the intravenous technique, and the dilution of the contrast material by the time it reaches the bladder is considerable. Therefore, when the urinary bladder is the focus of the examiner's attention, a retrograde technique is ordinarily employed. Retrograde cystography may be done simply by the introduction of an ordinary soft rubber catheter into the urinary bladder, followed by the retrograde instillation of undiluted contrast material under gravity pressure. Filling proceeds until the bladder is distended; this point may be judged by the patient's symptoms or by very brief occasional glimpses of the degree of filling through the image amplified fluoroscope. The catheter may then be removed and appropriate films may then be exposed in whatever projections are necessary to display suspected abnormalities. The ureters insert into the bladder posterolaterally; therefore, oblique films are necessary to display adquately this area, a single anteroposterior film of the pelvis being incomplete as a study of the urinary bladder.

Retrograde cystography is selected as the examination of choice when retrograde cystoureteral reflux is being sought (Figure 50). Under these circumstances the bladder is permitted to fill in a retrograde manner through a catheter (gravity flow), and it is ordinarily unnecessary to record by films or by cinecystography the presence of ureteral reflux until maximal filling of the bladder has been obtained. After this has been done, films in the anteroposterior and in both oblique projections will display not only the morphology of the bladder but also of the ureters, ordinarily dilated and filled by reflux. Particularly important is the demonstration of the ureterovesical junction in order that intrinsic abnormalities may be sought at these points. The degree of hydronephrosis resulting from reflux and superimposed infection should also be recorded. Whether or not the

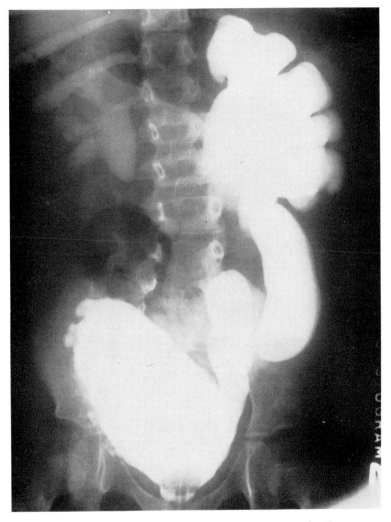

Figure 50. Reflux hydronephrosis (retrograde cystogram). Contrast material was introduced into the urinary bladder by means of a catheter. The bladder is enlarged and trabeculated, and reflux into the grossly dilated left ureter outlines the pronounced hydronephrosis and hydroureter on the left. The etiology was neurogenic.

dilated ureters display peristaltic activity should also be observed and if necessary, recorded by cinefluorography. A single film exposed following retrograde cystography and following the patient's attempt to completely empty the bladder will disclose potentially valuable information regarding the presence and volume of residual urine.

Retrograde cystography (and urethrography) should be routine in the study of the child with persistent or recurrent urinary tract infection. In this way, potentially correctable lesions which predispose to and perpetuate urinary tract infections may be discovered and properly treated.

URETHROGRAPHY

Radiologic inspection of the male or female urethra may be accomplished in several ways. Contrast material may be injected in a retrograde manner into the urethra, during which procedure films are exposed (Figure 51). Particularly valuable for such a technique is a thickened contrast substance, and there is commercially available a specially thickened 50% solution of sodium acetrizoate which is quite satisfactory (not for intravenous use!). The injection may be accomplished with a blunt syringe, and the contrast material is introduced slowly. Alternatively, the bladder may be filled with opaque material in a retrograde manner and voiding cystourethrography performed. This has become the method of choice in recent years. In this case an ordinary aqueous solution is employed, and sodium acetrizoate is commercially prepared in a 30% solution and in 250 ml bottles for that purpose (but not for intravenous injection).

The appearance of the contrast-filled urinary bladder and urethra during the act of voiding may be recorded radiologically in several ways. A single film may be exposed at the height of voiding with the patient turned obliquely, and in this way morphological details may be fairly well seen. Since the examination records the appearance of the bladder and urethra at only one short instant in time, some examiners have found this method unsatisfactory, and in general it has little to recommend it when methods of serial filming of the urethra are readily available. More satisfactory is the exposure of several films during the act of voiding; this may be done with an overhead tube and a device for manually changing films rapidly, or it may be done with a conventional spot film device under certain circumstances. More

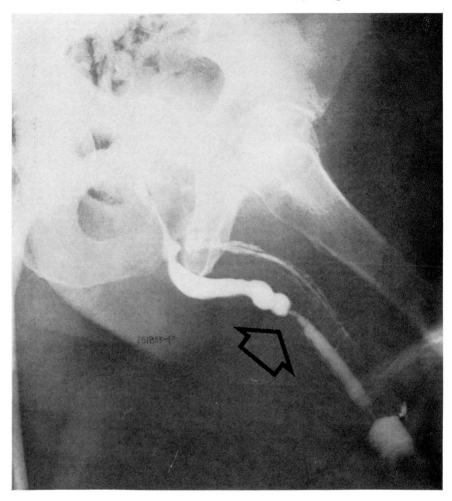

Figure 51. Urethral stricture (retrograde urethrogram). Contrast material was injected in a retrograde manner into the distal extremity of the penile urethra. The arrow points to a pronounced area of narrowing in the mid-portion of the pendulous urethra. The increased pressure associated with injection past such a tight stricture is responsible for the intravasation of contrast material into veins on the dorsum of the penis, seen as elongated strands of contrast material just superior to the opacified urethra.

satisfactory is the use of an automatic serial film changer which can expose as many films as desired at speeds of several exposures per second. Finally, cinecystourethrography provides a superior means of recording the fluoroscopic image permanently on film. Using such a technique, the mechanics of bladder contraction and emptying and the appearance of the urethra during urination can be recorded in considerable detail at film speeds of 15 to 30 frames per second. Ordinarily, very much slower speeds are acceptable, and 7.5 frames per second is usually quite adequate. Radiation exposure is considerably increased when cinefluorography is employed.

The patient is placed in an oblique position for voiding cystourethrography as for retrograde urethrography in order to demonstrate both the urethra and the bladder neck. The lateral position is also satisfactory, but the thickness of the pelvic structures and superimposition of bony parts in this view makes the oblique position generally more acceptable and satisfactory.

Urethrography is indicated in patients in whom suspicion of urinary tract obstruction in the vicinity of the bladder neck or more distal to that point is entertained. In patients suspected of having urethral strictures or stenoses, obstructing valves, fistulas, or sinuses, the examination is of value. On occasion, one will be able to demonstrate vesicoureteral reflux only during the act of voiding, and a voiding cystourethrogram is an important means of searching for that abnormality when ordinary means are unsuccessful.

ABDOMINAL AORTOGRAPHY

Certain abnormalities of the urinary tract are best studied by examination of films which display the vascular anatomy of the part involved. Most often it is renal arteriography that is desired, though on occasions pelvic arteriography displaying the vascular supply of a neoplasm of the urinary bladder may be of value in staging and in planning therapy. Display of the renal arteries can ordinarily be accomplished quite satisfactorily by injection of contrast material into the abdominal aorta. Aortography is preferably performed by the retrograde catheter approach, and the catheter may be introduced either into the femoral artery or into the left brachial or axillary artery. Under fluoroscopic control the catheter is positioned at or slightly distal to the origin of the renal arteries (when the approach is from below), and 20 to 30 ml of contrast material are injected, using a power injection (an adequate volume of contrast material cannot be delivered in a sufficiently short time by hand in most instances). Serial films are exposed at the rate of two to four per second centered over the kidneys. After inspection of the films, if it is determined that the examination has been satisfactory and additional injections are not required, the catheter is gently removed and pressure held over the point of puncture for several minutes until hemostasis is assured. The examination is performed under local anesthesia; in the hands of an experienced operator, complications are unusual. In some institutions abdominal aortography for study of the renal arteries is performed by the translumbar route. Versatility with such a technique is low, and a very much less satisfactory examination is likely to be obtained.

Abdominal aortography is indicated in several kinds of conditions. It is of particular value in suspected lesions of the renal arteries. Atherosclerotic renal artery stenosis and occlusion may be well demonstrated by such a technique, as well as the collateral blood supply to the kidney which may develop in such circumstances from ureteral, adrenal, lumbar and other arteries arising from the aorta. Fibromuscular hyperplasia of the renal arteries may also be well displayed, as may the stenoses associated with Takayasu's arteritis and homocystinuria. Aneurysms of the renal arteries are susceptible to demonstration by retrograde catheter abdominal aortography, and obstructions to small peripheral renal arteries may be demonstrated as may segmental infarction of the kidney. The latter can be surmised from the presence of wedge-shaped radiolucent defects in the nephrogram seen on the later films in the series. Suspected renal anomalies may be studied by abdominal aortography. Demonstration of the blood supply to a horseshoe kidney or a pelvic kidney may be important prior to surgical therapy, and aortography may be valuable in locating aberrant vessels producing ureteropelvic junction obstruction.

Abdominal aortography for the study of lesions of the kidneys has proven to be of special value in suspected mass lesions. The arteriographic appearance of a benign avascular cyst of the kidney is characteristic, showing vessels stretched around the smooth border of the lesion and showing a discrete rounded radiolucent defect on the nephrogram. In contrast, malignant neoplasms of the kidney commonly show wildly branching and exceedingly bizarre and unusual vessels supplying the tumor, vessels which are increased in number, abnormal in caliber, and which often show numerous arteriovenous shunts. No radiolucent defect is found in the nephrographic phase. It is true that some malignant neoplasms of the kidney have a sparse blood supply, but these are unusual, and careful search will ordinarily disclose the presence of tumor vessels. The coexistence of renal cyst and tumor in the same kidney is very unusual (1% of 1,007 consecutive cases of surgically proved renal cysts or tumors at the Mayo Clinic in a recent report), and abdominal aortography for study of the renal arteries should permit distinction to be made between these two lesions in the overwhelming majority of cases.

Finally, abdominal aortography should be performed prior to operations in which a donor kidney is substituted for a failing kidney, in the recipient to establish the vascular anatomy prior to operation and in the donor to determine the number of arteries, the status of the kidney in question, and particularly the status of the remaining kidney.

SELECTIVE RENAL ARTERIOGRAPHY

On occasion, injection of contrast material through a catheter placed in the abdominal aorta will provide inadequate opacification of the renal vascularity and parenchyma, particularly when careful examination of minute detail is required. In such circumstances and perhaps regularly in the study of cysts and tumors, selective renal arteriography may be employed (Figures 52 and 53). A specially curved catheter is introduced percutaneously and advanced to the level of the renal arteries where the one or ones in question may be selectively catheterized. By hand, 8 to 10 ml of contrast material are injected, during and following which serial films are exposed. Exquisite portrayal of the renal arteries is regularly obtained in this way, and delayed films show an excellent nephrogram. The renal vein is often well seen on films exposed four to ten seconds after injection. Immediately following the injection the catheter is withdrawn into the ab-

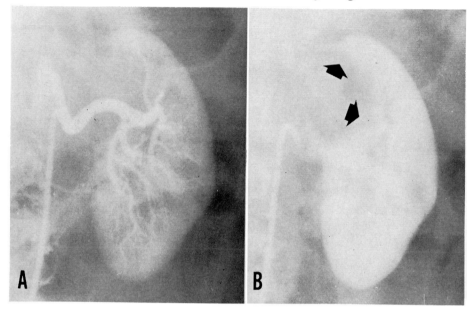

Figure 52. Benign renal cyst (selective renal arteriogram). (A) The arterial phase shows no evidence of tumor vessels and a sizable area of diminished vascularity on the medial aspect of the superior pole of the left kidney. (B) In the nephrogram phase one sees a smooth radiolucent defect in the upper pole representing the benign renal cyst. The remainder of the parenchyma is densely opaque.

dominal aorta to allow free flow of blood to the kidney, and if the films are satisfactory, the examination is terminated in the usual manner. A second injection is permissible if needed, and whatever projection is required may be used.

The increasing trend toward early application of renal arteriography to the solution of properly selected diagnostic problems is justified by the high yield of valuable information that can be obtained. With experience, the examination can be performed quickly and safely; correct interpretation also requires experience, and the study should not be undertaken by the occasional arteriographer.

RENAL VENOGRAPHY

Opacification of the renal veins for diagnostic purposes may be done in several ways. A catheter may be introduced percutaneously into a femoral vein and advanced into the inferior

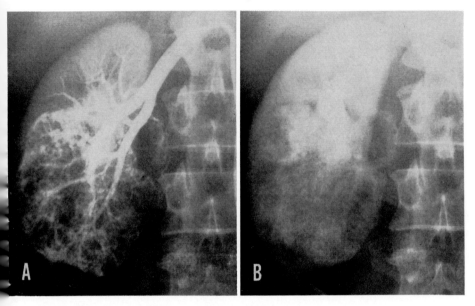

Figure 53. Carcinoma of the kidney (selective renal arteriogram). (A) The lower two thirds of the right kidney has been converted into an irregular hypervascular tumor mass, containing numerous areas of increased vascularity which are decidedly different than the normal vascularity to the upper pole. (B) In the nephrographic phase the tumor is seen as interspersed areas of increased and diminished density, but there is no smooth clean-cut radiolucent defect such as one sees with a benign renal cyst.

vena cava, where its tip is positioned opposite the expected entrance of the renal veins. Contrast material is injected while the patient performs an intense Valsalva maneuver, and reflux of contrast material into the renal veins may occur which can then be recorded on films. This is a very much less than satisfactory method of demonstrating the renal veins. More successful is the placement of a curved catheter directly into the renal vein on one or both sides, followed by the injection of contrast material and serial filming. A more direct approach to the renal veins which does not require the passage of a catheter through their vena caval orifices is by translumbar puncture of the kidney with a long needle, followed by gentle aspiration as the needle is withdrawn until venous blood is obtained. Contrast material is then injected directly into the intrarenal portions of the renal vein, and venography performed.

The indications for renal venography are few. Thrombosis of the renal vein may be studied in this way, but one may question the safety of introducing a catheter directly into the orifice of the renal vein from the vena cava when that orifice may be filled with clot, and one may inadvertently dislodge a thrombus which will lodge in the lungs. In such cases it may be sufficient to inject into the lower part of the inferior vena cava and demonstrate the thrombus in the renal vein protruding into the vena cava. The percutaneous transrenal approach to renal venography is a satisfactory alternative but has been tested to only a limited degree in humans.

Another indication for renal venography is the study of tumors of the kidney in which information regarding invasion of the renal vein by the neoplasm is desired. This information can frequently be obtained by injecting a slightly larger volume of contrast material at the time of selective renal arteriography, the delayed films then showing the renal veins satisfactorily. When this is impossible, catheterization of the renal vein may be employed, but one again risks laceration of tumor projecting into the renal vein by the catheter.

Finally, renal venography has been used in the study of renovascular hypertension. A catheter is introduced into the renal vein, contrast material is injected under standardized conditions, and renal cinevenography is performed. The renal venous washout time reflects the rate of blood flow through the kidney and is related to the presence of significant renal artery stenosis and to the renal plasma flow.

INFERIOR VENACAVOGRAPHY

Contrast opacification of the inferior vena cava is a simple and valuable special procedure for study of the effects of retroperitoneal tumors, some of which encroach upon and obstruct the vena cava (Figure 54). It is also valuable for study of the extent of the lesion in suspected renal vein and vena caval thrombosis. The examination may be performed very simply by the introduction of a needle or catheter into each femoral vein, followed by the simultaneous injection of contrast material on

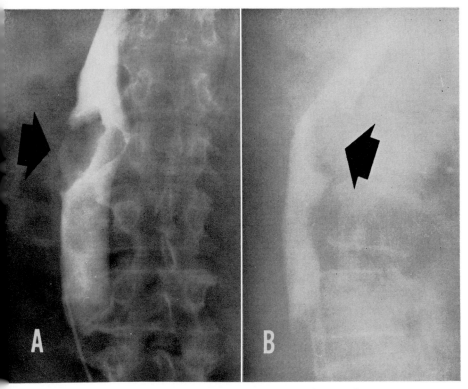

Figure 54. Carcinoma of the kidney with spread into the vena cava. Frontal (A) and lateral (B) films from a serial sequence following opacification of the inferior vena cava by injection through a catheter placed there through one femoral vein shows lobulated radiolucent defects within the lumen which represent direct extension from a carcinoma of the kidney. The tumor reached the vena caval lumen by way of the renal vein.

each side and serial filming over the abdomen in frontal and lateral projections. On each side, 25 to 30 ml may be injected. If a catheter is introduced into the distal part of the inferior vena cava and a single injection made, 40 to 50 ml will generally prove adequate. Films should be made in both frontal and lateral positions to assess the effect of retroperitoneal neoplasms upon the vena cava, and it is well to expose the lateral films first in order that the pyelogram which always results following the first injection will not obscure the vena cava on lateral films made following the anterposterior series. Retroperitoneal tumors which encroach upon or invade the vena cava will generally be found to be inoperable at surgery. There is, of course, no guarantee that those renal and other retroperitoneal tumors which do not produce a perceptible effect upon the opacified vena cava will be resectable. In general, it has been our experience that inferior venacavography is more valuable than renal arteriography in determining the resectability of renal neoplasms.

RETROPERITONEAL PNEUMOGRAPHY

The procedures thus far described have been designed for the most part to demonstrate the internal structure of the kidney collecting system or vascular tree. It is true that in several of these studies a nephrogram is obtained which allows inspection of the outer surface of the kidney. When greater contrast between the renal parenchyma and the surrounding structures is desired in order to delineate the size and shape of renal, adrenal, or other retroperitoneal masses or to localize the kidney prior to biopsy when renal function is too poor to permit excretory urography or isotope scanning, retroperitoneal gas insufflation may be employed. Carbon dioxide is commonly used for this purpose, and the gas may be introduced either by the more classical presacral route or by translumbar needles, one on each side, the tips of which lie adjacent to the kidney in the retroperitoneal fat. After introduction of the gas under local anesthesia, the patient may be turned into any of several positions, including the prone, supine, oblique and erect positions, to satisfactorily display the retroperitoneal gross anatomy. When the procedure is employed for the study of the adrenal glands when tumor is suspected, the presacral rather than the translumbar route should be employed. An occasional complicated and difficult-to-diagnose problem may require the combination of several of the procedures previously mentioned in addition to retroperitoneal pneumography, and such combined procedures are often valuable in accurate delineation of retroperitoneal masses. The combination of retroperitoneal gas insufflation with excretory urography and nephrotomography is a particularly valuable one.

PUNCTURE AND ASPIRATION OF RENAL CYSTS

On occasion, the differential diagnosis of renal cysts and tumors may require the puncture of a cystic lesion of the kidney with aspiration and analysis of the cyst contents. Under fluoroscopic control after opacification of the renal collecting systems following intravenous injection of an appropriate contrast material, a needle may be introduced through the back and into the cyst. Aspiration of fluid and its analysis for fat content and tumor cells may assist in the differential diagnosis, and the demonstration of the cyst wall by a double contrast technique utilizing air and contrast material introduced through the puncturing needle may add to the definitive assessment of such lesions. The inner surface of a benign cyst will ordinarily be quite smooth and have a very thin wall, while a cystic or necrotic neoplasm will have a thicker and much more irregular inner surface The examination is no more complex, difficult or hazardous than translumbar aortography, and it can be performed without undue discomfort or risk to the patient.

Chapter 9

THE REPRODUCTIVE SYSTEM

THE MALE

The Prostate Gland

PLAIN FILMS OF THE MALE PELVIS are ordinarily exposed exclusively in the frontal projection, usually a supine anteroposterior film. Prostatic calculi, indicating the presence of chronic prostatitis, are seen as ordinarily multiple and usually very small but quite dense stones superimposed upon the upper part of the symphysis pubis. Their small size, location and number will help the examiner exclude bladder stones. Other abnormalities of the prostate ordinarily have no radiologic manifestation in the prostate gland itself.

Carcinoma of the prostate commonly metastasizes to bone. Plain films of the part of the skeletal system involved are adequate to display the extent and ordinarily the nature of the abnormality. About the only serious differential diagnostic problem is Paget's disease. Metastases from carcinoma of the prostate are usually sclerotic but are commonly mixed lytic and productive lesions. Paget's disease, on the other hand, produces coarsened trabeculae, thickened cortex, and commonly, enlargement of the involved bone.

Osteitis pubis is best displayed on a frontal film of the pelvis and may occur following prostatectomy in males. The appearance is that of a mixed sclerotic and lytic lesion, usually on the superior margin of the pubis adjacent to the symphysis. It may be due to a smouldering, indolent, low-grade infection.

The only contrast examination of any practical value in examination of the prostate is cystourethrography. Prostatic enlargement is seen in the contrast-filled bladder as extrinsic filling defects, sometimes lobulated, on the inferior aspect of the bladder (Figure 55). An enlarged prostate may also elevate and deform

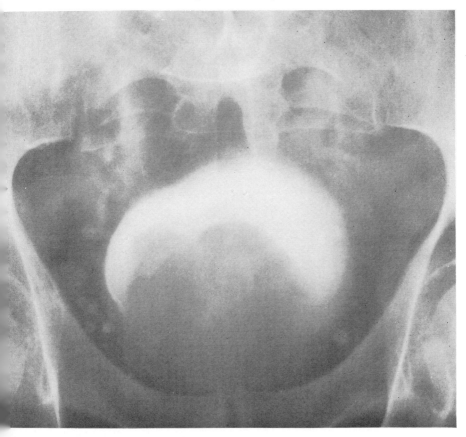

Figure 55. Benign prostatic hypertrophy (excretory urogram). The bladder has been rendered opaque by intravenous injection of contrast material, and on its undersurface is seen a large lobulated radiolucent defect representing the greatly enlarged prostate gland. It is impossible to distinguish benign hypertrophy from carcinoma of the prostate by observation of the filling defect alone.

the bladder. If the enlargement is sharply localized, the spurious appearance of a filling defect within the lumen of the bladder may be seen. The urethra may be constricted and deformed by prostatic enlargement, and infection with fistulous tracts may be visualized by contrast studies of the urethra. When prostatic carcinoma is invasive and involves the bladder or urethra, deformities resulting from this invasion may be visible.

Seminal Vesicles

The only plain film finding indicative of an abnormality of the seminal vesicles is calcification. The shape and location are usually characteristic and leave no doubt as to the organ involved. The calcification is ordinarily the consequence of old infection resulting from gonorrhea or tuberculosis.

Seminal vesiculography is rarely performed. The reflux of contrast material into the seminal vesicles following injection into the vas deferens on either side may produce opacification sufficient to permit the diagnosis of strictures, stenoses, cavitation, and irregular deformity secondary to infection. Distention of the urethra with contrast substance rarely fills the seminal vesicles by reflux.

Calcification in the Vas Deferens

This is commonly associated with diabetes mellitus. The vasa deferentia may be opacified by injection near the origin of the vas deferens in the spermatic cord. Areas of irregularity, stenosis or unusual dilatation, ordinarily a result of infection, may be displayed thereby. The examination is rarely performed.

The Urethra

Plain films may show stones lying within urethral diverticula, but the plain film examination is rarely of value otherwise.

Numerous techniques are available for contrast opacification of the male urethra. Intravenously injected contrast substance may be allowed to collect in the urinary bladder, following which the patient voids while films are exposed. More satisfactory is the retrograde filling of the bladder by means of a catheter, following which the catheter is removed and the patient voids, thus rendering the urethra opaque. A thick jellylike contrast-impregnated material may also be introduced retrograde in the urethra, and this permits distention of the urethra and allows the exposure of numerous static films.

Filming may be accomplished in a number of ways: (a) conventional still films, (b) serial films and (c) cinefluorography.

The abnormalities susceptible to display by urethrography include the following: bladder neck obstruction from any cause, congenital urethral valves and septa, stenoses and strictures, sinus tracts and fistulas, diverticula, abscesses, polyps, tumors, and mucosal irregularity secondary to infection, often granulomatous.

THE FEMALE

Plain Films

Soft tissue masses of many sorts may be visualized as more or less well circumscribed opacities of water density in the pelvis and lower abdomen. The most common normal structures to produce such findings are a full bladder and a pregnant uterus. The most common abnormalities to produce such opacities are uterine leiomyomas and ovarian cysts. Most often, pelvic tumors and cysts which arise from the female generative apparatus are not radiographically distinguishable from one another. At times they contain calcifications which permit prediction of the organ of origin. The irregular popcornlike calcifications seen with uterine leiomyomas are an example of such calcifications, but they may take almost any form (Figure 56). When very dense and discrete calcifications are seen within a pelvic soft tissue mass, particularly when they have a form suggesting bone or teeth, ovarian teratoma may be diagnosed with a high degree of accuracy. Teratomas commonly contain collections of oily sebaceous material which may appear relatively radiolucent in one area of the soft tissue mass.

Phleboliths, calculi within pelvic veins, are often seen on ordinary films of the pelvis in women. They are distinguished by their multiplicity (usually) and by the fact that most of them contain a tiny radiolucent dot generally asymmetrically situated within the calcium deposit. They are of no clinical significance but may occasionally be of value in diagnosis. The demonstration of a decided shift in the position of previously noted phleboliths in a woman with a pelvic tumor suggests enlargement and spread of the neoplasm.

Plain films may show the presence of foreign bodies in the pelvis. Pessaries and diaphragms with opaque rims will be visible in the vagina, and most intrauterine contraceptive devices are visible in the uterus, though some are more opaque than others.

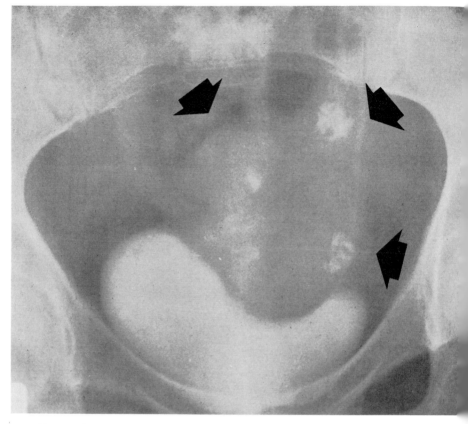

Figure 56. Uterine leiomyomas (excretory urogram). A lobulated soft tissue mass (arrows) indents the dome of the bladder and contains some popcorn-like calcifications characteristic of uterine fibroids.

Intrauterine contraceptive devices may erode their way out of the uterus and into the peritoneal cavity where they may also be seen on plain films, often in unusual locations. Other foreign bodies may be found in the vagina and uterus, such as hairpins, paper clips, bits of wire, and so on.

Plain films of the abdomen have been used for years to localize the placenta. Films in frontal and lateral projections are obtained, usually with the patient in the erect position. The placental location is inferred from the soft tissue opacity which it casts as well as the displacement of the fetus in a direction opposite the location of the placenta. Compression devices have been used to enhance the ability of the observer to see the placenta, and in the hands of those experienced in its use, the plain film examination may be very accurate. Most have abandoned it and now prefer some means of directly opacifying the placenta. When the placenta is partly calcified, it may be easily located on plain films.

Conventional films of the abdomen and pelvis have many uses in obstetrics. The skeleton of a fetus ordinarily becomes visible at about fourteen to twenty weeks of pregnancy, and the fact of pregnancy may thereby be confirmed (though there are better ways!). More often, radiographic studies of the pregnant abdomen are employed in a search for the cause of failure of the presenting part to progress during labor. A standing lateral film of the pelvis may be of special value under such circumstances and may show that the cause is an abnormality in fetal position or presentation. Less often, the cause will be found to be an abnormality of the fetus, such as hydrocephalus. Film studies will not always disclose the cause of failure of labor to progress, especially when the cause is some deficiency in the expulsive power of the uterus or when a soft tissue mass without calcification partly obstructs the outlet.

Other fetal abnormalities may be diagnosed with relative ease by conventional films of the abdomen in pregnancy. Anencephaly may be diagnosed with certainty (Figure 57), as may certain other kinds of monstrosity in which the skeleton is affected. Multiple pregnancies may be disclosed by plain films of the abdomen, and such studies may be requested when that diagnosis is suspected. Current obstetrical thought advocates prolonged bed rest for women bearing more than one fetus in an effort to diminish the prematurity and neonatal mortality rate. Confirmation of the presence of a multiple pregnancy may thus have important therapeutic and prognostic implications.

A missed abortion may sometimes be found unexpectedly on plain films of the abdomen, particularly when the fetal death occurred years before. The skeleton of the fetus may be clearly visible, though it is often deformed. At times, an abdominal pregnancy will result in death of the fetus with the subsequent

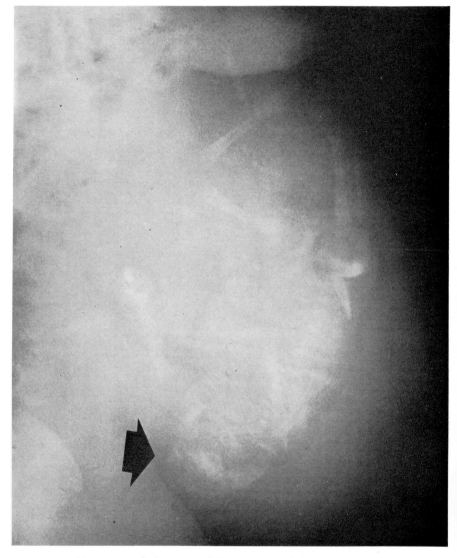

Figure 57. Anencephaly. Lateral film of the abdomen of this pregnant woman shows the presence of a well-developed late third trimester fetus. Only the bones of the base of the skull have developed (arrow), and no calvarium is present in this anencephalic monstrosity. Anencephaly is commonly associated with polyhydramnios.

formation of a lithopedion, and a partly calcified sac containing parts of a fetal skeleton may be visualized radiographically.

Plain films of the abdomen are also employed for pelvimetry, and such films usually have a measuring device of some sort included by means of which magnification may be taken into consideration. The pelvic diameters may be measured and compared with normal, and an estimation of the ease with which the fetus will pass through the birth canal may be obtained. Deformities of the maternal pelvis which may impede labor or prevent delivery from below may also be recognized. The examination is indicated when manual abdominal and pelvic examinations are thought insufficient to allow a decision to be made regarding the possibility of uncomplicated vaginal delivery.

Films of the abdomen and pelvis are also employed during pregnancy for the prediction of fetal maturity. Visualization of the distal femoral epiphyseal ossification centers on a film of the maternal abdomen is almost always associated with physiological maturity (capacity for independent, uncomplicated extrauterine life), and if both the distal femoral and proximal tibial epiphyseal ossification centers are seen, physiological maturity may be predicted with nearly 100 percent confidence. Other parameters may be employed for the prediction of fetal maturity. The lumbar spine may be measured and correlated with length of gestation and fetal length and age by appropriate tables, and the size of the fetal head may also be used to estimate maturity. The usual indications for exposure of films to evaluate fetal maturity include Rh incompatibility, eclampsia or preeclampsia, and other conditions in which either the fetal or maternal health would be threatened by continuing the pregnancy.

Radiologic signs of fetal death ordinarily require only plain films of the abdomen for adequate demonstration. Most reliable is gas within the fetal circulatory system (Figure 58). Signs of collapse of the fetal skull are also of a high order of reliability. Hyperflexion of the fetal spine suggests collapse of the fetal skeleton and fetal death, but foreshortening of a normal spine may give the spurious appearance of collapse (the fetal spine is ordinarily extended during uterine contractions during labor). Bizarre arrangements of fetal small parts suggest fetal death, as

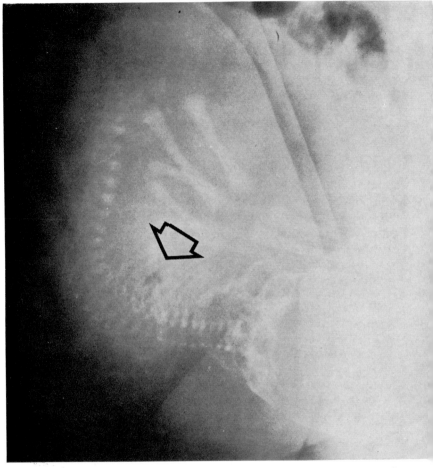

Figure 58. Fetal death. A lateral compression film of the abdomen shows the fetus to good advantage. The spine has assumed a hyper-flexed position, and there is some overlapping of the fetal skull bones. More impressive as a sign of fetal death is the presence of gas within the fetal heart (arrow).

does failure of the fetus to move from its position over a period of hours or days.

Overriding of the sutures of the skull suggests fetal death, but some degree of overriding of the fetal skull bones may be seen during normal labor, and the diagnosis must be made cautiously from such evidence. In general, unless the signs of fetal death are quite conclusive, film studies serve as confirmatory evidence of the clinical suspicion that the baby is dead.

Mammography

Soft tissue films of the breasts (without contrast material) display the cutaneous and internal (adipose, acinar, ductal, fibrous and vascular) anatomy of the breasts in considerable detail. The examination is utilized by many physicians as an aid in screening asymptomatic middle-aged and older women for carcinoma of the breast. It is also indicated in patients with breast masses when the diagnosis or therapy is in doubt and to help in examination of the "normal" breast in a patient with a tumor on the opposite side.

Films of the breasts are difficult to interpret, but certain lesions have characteristic if not diagnostic appearances. Carcinomas may show thickening of the skin, increased vascularity, a mass with irregular margins (Figures 59 and 60), and tiny, punctate calcifications. Benign lesions are generally more sharply circumscribed and may be densely calcified or multiple. Skillfully interpreted, mammography adds considerably to the diagnostic accuracy of the physical examination.

Excretory Urography and Cystography

The urinary tract may be profoundly affected by changes in the internal female genitalia. Ureteral obstruction may be produced by pressure from tumors and cysts in the pelvis, and the ureters may be obstructed by invasion from malignant neoplasms, especially carcinoma of the cervix. Urinary tract obstruction may also be the consequence of operative misadventure, with ligation or transection of one or both ureters. In this regard, it is sensible to obtain an excretory urogram prior to pelvic operations as a control study, facilitating the diagnosis of obstruction postoperatively should it occur.

Physiological hydronephrosis of pregnancy may be mistaken for pathological urinary tract obstruction by the observer who is unaware of its occurrence. The cause has been debated, but the best evidence supports the view that the hydronephrosis is the consequence of ureteral obstruction from an enlarged uterus. The

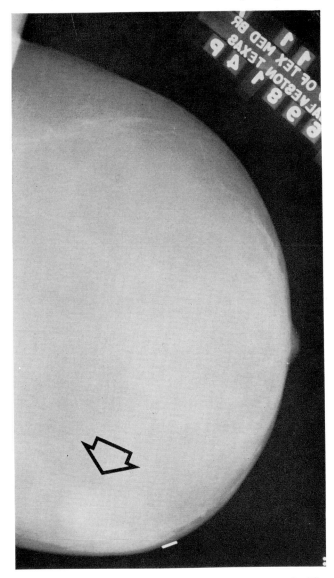

Figure 59. Carcinoma of the breast (ordinary mammogram). The medio-lateral view of the right breast shows the presence of a poorly defined soft tissue opacity outlined by fat which has largely replaced the parenchyma (arrow). The lesion is associated with some thickening of the adjacent skin. A dominant mass with skin thickening strongly suggests carcinoma.

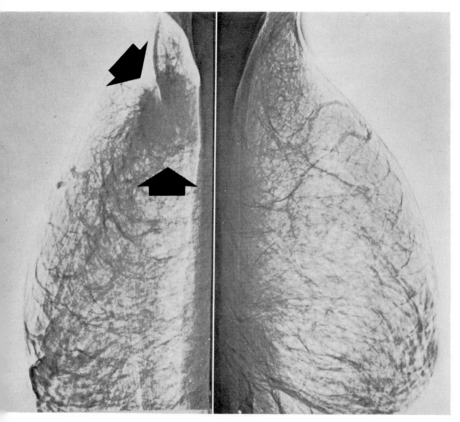

Figure 60. Carcinoma of the breast (xero-mammography). Arrows point to a mass lesion in the breast with spiculated margins indicating invasion of the adjacent tissues. The opposite breast is included for comparison and is normal. Detail of the breast tissues and ability to detect carcinoma is considerably improved by the xero-radiographic technique.

right side is ordinarily more affected than the left, and the dilatation of the collecting structures may last for weeks following delivery, gradually returning to normal. Because of the regular occurrence of dilatation of the urinary tract in the third trimester of pregnancy, it is wise to postpone elective diagnostic radiographic procedures on the urinary tract until four to six weeks following delivery in order that any abnormalities detected can be correctly attributed to some pathologic abnormality and not to the effects of pregnancy.

Back and flank discomfort, urinary frequency, and sometimes, dysuria are common symptoms late in pregnancy. If objective evidence of urinary tract infection is found but the patient fails to respond to appropriate medical therapy, or if symptoms are very severe and suggest the passage of a stone or obstruction secondary thereto, excretory urography may be performed during pregnancy. It is sensible to employ as few films as possible under these circumstances in order to limit the radiation exposure to both mother and fetus.

Excretory urography may show displacement of the kidneys, ureters or bladder resulting from pelvic masses of any sort. It is well to remember that not all pelvic masses in women are due to tumors of the genital apparatus, though most are (if one excludes full bladders and pregnant uteruses). Neoplasms of the colon or even of the small intestine, periappendiceal abscesses, anterior meningoceles, and anteriorly directed tumors of the skeleton may also produce pelvic masses which displace the urinary tract.

Cystography may be employed as an aid in placental localization as long as certain important limitations are borne in mind. The bladder may be rendered visible by introducing opaque material into it, or air or some other gas may be used. If the presenting part of the fetus is closely applied to the distended urinary bladder in both frontal and lateral projections, it is very unlikely that a low-lying placenta is present anteriorly. If the head of the fetus is separated from the urinary bladder, particularly if the separation is asymmetrical, anteriorly located low-lying placenta may be suspected. Diagnostic problems arise when third-trimester bleeding prompts the performance of cystography and no abnormality is found. A *posteriorly* located low-lying placenta or overt placenta previa may be present without distortion of the urinary bladder. For that reason, cystography is not recommended as a means of placental localization.

Barium Enema

The rectum and sigmoid may be displaced, distorted or invaded by tumors or cysts arising from the female genitalia. The sigmoid is usually smoothly draped over uterine leiomyomas or ovarian cysts, but the colon may be invaded and distorted in a bizarre way by carcinomas of the female genital organs which are metastatic to the rectum or sigmoid. Endometriosis occasionally involves the colon and may similarly distort the lumen by extrinsic pressure from nodules located beneath the mucosa.

An important cause of rectosigmoid abnormalities demonstrable by barium enema is radiation proctitis or colitis following radiation therapy for malignant neoplasms of the pelvis. Diagnostic difficulties occasionally arise in distinguishing between radiation effects and recurrence of a previously present and treated malignant neoplasm.

Hysterosalpingography

Opacification of the interior of the uterus and uterine tubes may be accomplished in many ways, some of which require the gynecologist's participation and some do not. Some methods utilize fluoroscopy, others only plain films. The method chosen depends largely upon personal preference and experience, and many variations are satisfactory.

The most common indication for hysterosalpingography is infertility. The hysterosalpingogram is performed in a search for structural abnormalities which prevent conception. Such abnormalities include congenital anomalies, unusual septa and synechiae, polyps and tumors within the lumen of the uterus, infantile uterus, and stenosis or obstruction of the uterine tubes. It is the last-named finding which is usually sought and which may present a formidable impediment to conception. In the presence of hydrosalpinx or pyosalpinx, the contrast material fills a dilated clubbed uterine tube, and spill of the contrast material into the peritoneal cavity is not seen.

Some previously infertile women become pregnant after sexual intercourse following hysterosalpingography. This usually diagnostic procedure may thus occasionally have therapeutic value, though the precise mechanism is unknown. Perhaps tiny filmy adhesions are eliminated by the passage of the contrast material through the uterine tubes.

Hysterosalpingography is also valuable in the study of other suspected abnormalities of the uterus and tubes. Endometrial hyperplasia of whatever cause produces nodular irregularities of the margins of the contrast column within the uterus. Polyps and submucosal and intramural leiomyomas may project into the uterine lumen as filling defects or greatly deform the wall (Figure 61). Some polyps and fibroids may actually project through the cervical canal. Carcinoma of the uterus may be seen on films following the introduction of contrast material into the uterus, but a woman bleeding from the uterus or with an enlarged uterus because of a pelvic mass is more likely to have an operation (such as a curettement) than a hysterosalpingogram. Moreover,

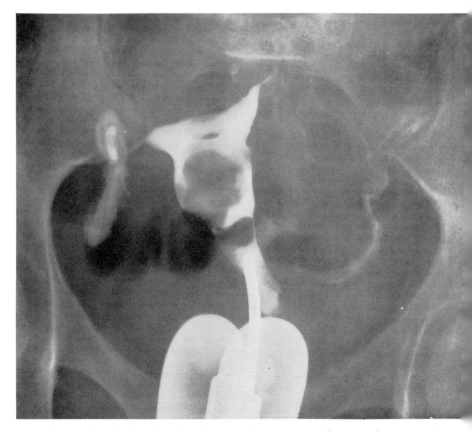

Figure 61. Pedunculated submucous leiomyomas (hysterosalpingogram). Contrast material has been introduced into the uterus, and it fills both uterine tubes. Within the uterine cavity are one large and one small lobulated radiolucent filling defect, both of which were found to represent pedunculated submucosal leiomyomas. Endometrial polyps would have the same appearance.

there is the danger of intravasation of the contrast material in a patient with carcinoma of the endometrium, and it is at least theoretically possible to drive malignant cells into the venous or lymphatic circulation by the procedure, particularly if the intra-uterine pressure is elevated.

Intrauterine and tubal pregnancy may be demonstrated by hysterosalpingography, but every effort is made not to perform such an examination if the patient is thought to be pregnant or at a time when the patient could be pregnant. Thus, hystero-salpingography is ordinarily scheduled for the first two weeks following the start of a normal menstrual period in order to be certain that the examination is not performed upon a pregnant woman. There is one circumstance in which hysterosalpingogra-phy may be indicated in the presence of a known pregnancy. That is when an ectopic pregnancy is suspected. A hystero-salpingogram showing an empty uterus of normal size establishes the diagnosis.

Hydrosalpinx as the cause of a pelvic mass and as the source of a patient's symptoms may be demonstrated by hysterosal-pingography. So may chronic infections which do not necessarily produce hydrosalpinx. Tuberculous endometritis may produce both hyperplasia of the endometrium and ulceration with tiny sinus tracts, particularly in the endocervical canal, diagnosable by hysterosalpingography.

Congenital abnormalities of the female pelvic viscera which are susceptible to display by this modality are largely variations of bicornuate uterus. One may see anything from a tiny residual septum in the fundus to a complete uterus didelphys.

Diagnostic Pelvic Pneumoperitoneum

Gas is introduced into the pelvic peritoneal cavity in any one of a number of ways, and the patient is positioned so that the gas is trapped in the pelvic cavity (head down, pelvis up). Films are exposed using a technique which emphasizes soft tissue rather than bony detail. Any rapidly absorbed gas is acceptable; carbon dioxide and nitrous oxide are usually used. The gas may be introduced through the abdominal wall (the usual way) or through the cervical canal, from which point it finds access to the peritoneal cavity through the uterine tubes.

Such a study shows the peritonealized surfaces of the female pelvic organs. The dome of the bladder is seen, as are the uterus, uterine tubes, ovaries and round ligaments. Lesions which distort the external surfaces of these organs are plainly visible, even as lesions which distort the internal or luminal surface are visible by hysterosalpingography. Diagnostic pelvic pneumoperitoneum is indicated particularly in women in whom ordinary bimanual pelvic examination is difficult or contraindicated. Most often, the indication will be suspected pelvic pathology in an obese woman, but the examination may also be employed in children and in women with vaginal or cervical abnormalities which preclude a satisfactory pelvic examination. One of the advantages of diagnostic pelvic pneumoperitoneum over the standard manual pelvic examination is the ability of more than one person to observe pelvic abnormalities simultaneously, an impossibility with the usual pelvic examination. There is no doubt about what mass is being discussed, what its shape is, or what side it is on when looking at films from a pelvic pneumogram, and such disagreements and difficulties may at times arise with the ordinary pelvic examination.

Pelvic pneumography offers the possibility of obtaining information regarding the presence or absence of pelvic organs, their size, shape and location, and specific abnormalities may be displayed. Cysts and tumors may be outlined and localized. Enlarged multicystic ovaries found in the Stein-Leventhal syndrome may be clearly shown (Figure 62). Adhesions of the pelvic viscera to the intestine may be displayed, and tubal enlargement and deformity such as is seen with hydrosalpinx or ectopic pregnancy may be shown. Congenital anomalies which produce deformities of the external surface of the pelvic organs may be shown, examples of which are bicornuate uterus and congenital absence of the uterus, perhaps with rudimentary uterine horns seen laterally on either pelvic wall.

Pelvic Arteriography

Opacification of the arteries of the pelvis, ordinarily by the retrograde femoral catheter route, is employed almost exclusively for the study of tumors and cysts of the female genital tract and

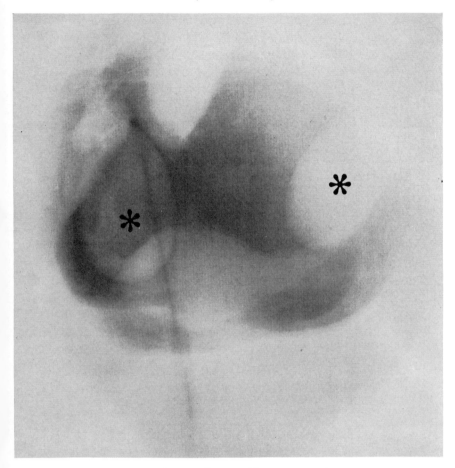

Figure 62. Stein-Leventhal syndrome (diagnostic pelvic pneumoperitoneum). Carbon dioxide has been introduced into the pelvic peritoneal cavity and outlines the peritonealized surfaces of the internal female generative organs. The asterisks mark the smoothly and symmetrically enlarged ovaries, and the soft tissue opacity between them is the uterus. Each ovary is as large as the uterus, a distinctly abnormal condition.

for placental localization. Trophoblastic tumors may produce characteristic arterial patterns and allow a specific diagnosis to be made. Choriocarcinoma is a very vascular neoplasm, containing large vascular lakes and pools and often demonstrating the presence of tumor vessels, tumor stain and early venous filling.

Hydatidiform mole, on the other hand, is usually avascular, the grapelike clusters of the tumor occupying the usually blood-filled intervillous spaces. Pelvic arteriography is rarely employed for the study of carcinoma of the cervix or of the endometrium, as neither is a notoriously vascular neoplasm. However, cervical carcinoma may on occasion show a tumor stain, and it may displace, invade, encase and even obstruct the pelvic arteries. Thus, pelvic arteriography may be particularly useful in a patient with carcinoma of the cervix, previously treated, in whom recurrence is suspected.

A properly timed film following the injection of contrast material into the distal abdominal aorta will opacify the placental venous sinusoids (intervillous spaces) and allow precise localization of the placenta. Only one film (in addition to a scout film for positioning and technique) is ordinarily necessary for such an examination. Different examiners depend upon different positions of the patient, some preferring the frontal view, others the lateral view, and still others an oblique view. Most use a catheter technique to inject the contrast agent into the distal abdominal aorta. A reliable intravenous technique has also been developed. The examination is highly reliable and exposes the patient and fetus to little radiation.

Pelvic Venography

The pelvic veins may be rendered opaque by injection of contrast material into each femoral vein, followed by filming in the frontal projection over the pelvis. Pelvic masses of any kind may displace or obstruct the veins of the pelvis, and malignant neoplasms may invade the pelvic veins. It is unusual for pelvic venography to be performed for the study of the effect of masses upon the venous system unless an extensive operation is anticipated and detailed knowledge of pelvic anatomy is necessary in advance.

Pelvic venous congestion and phlebitis are not often displayed by the usual method of pelvic venography, namely, injecting contrast material into the femoral veins. The pelvic veins ordinarily involved are those which form a plexus about the bladder and uterus, and these are not seen unless special injection techniques are employed. The contrast agent may be deposited directly into the cervical muscle, and veins and lymphatics draining the area may then be rendered opaque. Or, a catheter may be introduced into the femoral vein and the hypogastric vein or its branches selectively catheterized and then rendered opaque by retrograde injection. Neither of these techniques is commonly employed in diagnosis.

Lymphangiography

Lymphangiography is valuable for the staging of lymphomas, that is, to determine whether or not the pelvic and retroperitoneal lymph nodes are involved by a neoplasm known to be present elsewhere. It may also occasionally be of value in the diagnosis of metastases to lymph nodes from pelvic malignancies, but there is such a wide variation in the appearance of normal lymph nodes that the value of the procedure is limited. Pelvic infections at any time in the past may produce areas of fibrosis in lymph nodes indistinguishable from the defects produced by metastatic disease. When plainly and obviously positive, lymphangiograms in tumors other than lymphomas may be of value (seminoma, for example), but a negative study by no means excludes metastatic disease. Because lymph nodes remain opaque for long periods of time following lymphangiography, the spread of a pelvic malignancy may be followed by its effect in displacing as well as destroying opacified lymph nodes. The beneficial effects of surgical or radiation therapy may be monitored similarly.

Amniography

The removal of a small amount of amniotic fluid following transabdominal needle puncture of the amniotic cavity is no longer considered a hazardous procedure and may be extremely valuable in diagnosis. Neither is it hazardous to introduce contrast material into the amniotic cavity, shortly after which the entire volume of amniotic fluid becomes opaque. This may have value in the diagnosis of abnormalities of the fetus and of the mother. About the only maternal abnormality so demonstrated is polyhydramnios, and amniography is ordinarily not necessary for the purpose.

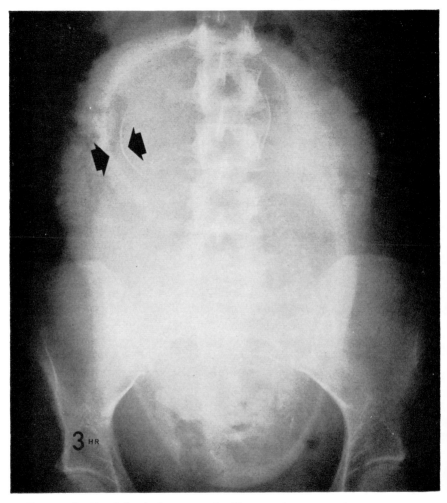

Figure 63. Fetal death due to erythroblastosis (amniogram). Contrast material was injected into the amniotic cavity three hours before this film was made. The integument of the fetus is visible between the arrows (the arrow on the left points to the outer surface of the skin and the arrow on the right points to the fetal skull). The skin thickness should not exceed about 4 millimeters, but in this hydropic edematous infant the scalp is much thickened. Also observe that in three hours none of the contrast material had passed into the fetal intestinal tract, a sign strongly suggestive of fetal death.

Hydrops fetalis may be suspected or even demonstrated by amniography when the edematous integument of the fetus can be shown (Figure 63). Thickening of the scalp, visible as a soft tissue opacity between the skull and the opacified amniotic fluid, is a strong clue to that diagnosis. Fetal death may also be diagnosed by amniography. A normal fetus ingests amniotic fluid continuously, and if the amniotic fluid is rendered opaque with contrast material, a film exposed several hours later will show the contrast material in the fetal alimentary canal. Failure to see the opacified gut under these circumstances is a suggestive sign of fetal death, but it is certainly not an absolute sign. Esophageal atresia may result in the same x-ray appearance. Other fetal abnormalities may also be shown to good advantage by amniography, and the sex of the unborn fetus may sometimes be predicted by visualization of the external aspect of the genitalia. The study is rarely performed for either of latter two purposes however.

Amniography is employed by some for placental localization. The placenta is indirectly visualized as a crescentic filling defect on one wall of the uterus.

Intrauterine fetal transfusion is performed by many obstetricians and radiologists without prior amniography, but some prefer to utilize the opacified intestinal tube of the fetus as a target for the needle through which the transfusion will subsequently be performed.

BIBLIOGRAPHY

GENERAL TEXTS

Caffey, John: *Pediatric X-ray Diagnosis*, 6th ed. Chicago, Year Book, 1972, 2 volumes.

Lasser, Elliott C.: *Dynamic Factors in Roentgen Diagnosis*. Baltimore, Williams and Wilkins, 1967.

Lusted, Lee B., and Keats, Theodore E.: *Atlas of Roentgenographic Measurement*, 3rd ed. Chicago, Year Book, 1972.

Meschan, Isadore: *Analysis of Roentgen Signs in General Radiology*. Philadelphia, Saunders, 1973, 2 volumes.

Paul, Lester W., and Juhl, John H.: *The Essentials of Roentgen Interpretation*, 3rd ed. New York, Harper & Row, 1972.

Potchen, E. James, Koehler, P. Ruben, and Davis, David O.: *Principles of Diagnostic Radiology*. New York, McGraw-Hill, 1971.

Schinz, H. R., Baensch, W. E., Frommhold, W., Glauner, R., Uehlinger, E., and Wellauer, J. (Eds.): *Roentgen Diagnosis*. New York, Grune and Stratton, 1968, 5 volumes.

Squire, Lucy Frank: *Fundamentals of Roentgenology*. Cambridge, Mass., Harvard University Press, 1964.

Sutton, David, and Grainger, Ronald (Eds.): *A Textbook of Radiology*. Edinburgh and London, E. and S. Livingstone Ltd., 1969.

Teplick, J. George, Haskin, Marvin E., and Schimert, Arnd P. (Eds.): *Roentgenologic Diagnosis (A Complement in Radiology to the Beeson and McDermott Textbook of Medicine)*. Philadelphia, Saunders, 1967, 2 volumes.

BONES

Aegerter, Ernest, and Kirkpatrick, John A., Jr.: *Orthopedic Diseases*. Philadelphia, Saunders, 1968.

Edeiken, Jack, and Hodes, Philip J.: *Roentgen Diagnosis of Diseases of Bone*. Baltimore, Williams and Wilkins, 1967.

Epstein, Bernard S.: *The Spine*. Philadelphia, Lea and Febiger, 1969.

Greenfield, George B.: *Radiology of Bone Diseases*. Philadelphia, Lippincott, 1969.

Lichtenstein, Louis: *Bone Tumors*. St. Louis, Mosby, 1959.

Murray, Ronald O., and Jacobson, Harold G.: *The Radiology of Skeletal Disorders*. Baltimore, Williams and Wilkins, 1971.

Rubin, Philip: *Dynamic Classification of Bone Dysplasias*. Chicago, Year Book, 1964.

165

Zimmer, E. A.: In Wilk, Stefan P. (Ed.): *Borderlands of the Normal and Early Pathologic in Skeletal Roentgenology.* New York, Grune and Stratton, 1968.

THE SKULL AND CENTRAL NERVOUS SYSTEM

di Chiro, Giovanni: *An Atlas of Detailed Normal Pneumoencephalographic Anatomy.* Springfield, Illinois, Thomas, 1961.

Du Boulay, G. H.: *Principles of X-ray Diagnosis of the Skull.* London, Butterworths, 1965.

Epstein, Bernard S.: *Pneumoencephalography and Cerebral Angiography.* Chicago, Year Book, 1966.

Etter, Lewis E.: *Atlas of Roentgen Anatomy of the Skull,* Rev. 3rd Ptg. Springfield, Illinois, Thomas, 1970.

Newton, Thomas H., and Potts, D. Gordon: *Radiology of the Skull and Brain.* St. Louis, Mosby, 1971, 3 volumes.

Shapiro, Robert: *Myelography.* Chicago, Year Book, 1968.

Taveras, Juan M., and Wood, Ernest H.: *Diagnostic Neuroradiology.* Baltimore, Williams and Wilkins, 1964.

Wilson, McClure: *The Anatomical Foundation of Neuroradiology of the Brain,* 2nd ed. Boston, Brown and Company, 1972.

THE URINARY TRACT

Emmett, John L., and Witten, David M.: *Clinical Urography,* 3rd ed. Philadelphia, Saunders, 1971, 3 volumes.

Flocks, Rubin H., Jonsson, Gosta, Lindblom, Knut, Olsson, Olle, Romanus, Ragnar, and Winter, Chester C.: *Encyclopedia of Urology, Diagnostic Radiology.* Berlin, Springer-Verlag, 1962, Vol. 1.

Kincaid, Owings W. (Ed.): *Renal Angiography.* Chicago, Year Book, 1966.

Ney, Charles, and Friedenberg, Richard M.: *Radiographic Atlas of the Genitourinary System.* Philadelphia, Lippincott, 1966.

The Radiologic Clinics of North America, Vol. III, No. 1, April 1965.

The Radiologic Clinics of North America, Vol. X, No. 3, December 1972.

THE CHEST

Felson, Benjamin: *Chest Roentgenology.* Philadelphia, Saunders, 1973.

———, Weinstein, Aaron S., and Spitz, Harold B.: *Principles of Chest Roentgenology.* Philadelphia, Saunders, 1965.

Fraser, Robert G., and Pare, J. A. Peter: *Diagnosis of Diseases of the Chest.* Philadelphia, Saunders, 1970, 2 volumes.

Leigh, Ted F., and Weens, H. Stephen: *The Mediastinum.* Springfield, Illinois, Thomas, 1959.

Seminars in Roentgenology, Vol. II, No. 1, January 1967; Vol. IV, No. 1, January 1969.

The Radiologic Clinics of North America, Vol. I, No. 2, August 1963.

THE HEART AND GREAT VESSELS

Cooley, Robert N., and Schreiber, Melvyn H.: *Radiology of the Heart and Great Vessels.* Baltimore, Williams and Wilkins, 1967.

Edwards, Jesse E.: *An Atlas of Acquired Diseases of the Heart and Great Vessels.* Philadelphia, Saunders, 1961, 3 volumes.

———, Carey, Lewis S., Neufeld, Henry N., and Lester, Richard G.: *Congenital Heart Disease.* Philadelphia, Saunders, 1965, 2 volumes.

Elliott, Larry P., and Schiebler, Gerald L.: *X-ray Diagnosis of Congenital Cardiac Disease.* Springfield, Illinois, Thomas, 1968.

Stewart, James R., Kincaid, Owings W., and Edwards, Jesse E.: *An Atlas of Vascular Rings and Related Malformations of the Aortic Arch System.* Springfield, Illinois, Thomas, 1964.

Taussig, Helen B.: *Congenital Malformations of the Heart.* Cambridge, Mass., Harvard University Press, 1960, 2 volumes.

The Radiologic Clinics of North America, Vol. IX, Nos. 2 and 3, August and December 1971.

THE ABDOMEN AND GASTROINTESTINAL TRACT

Margulis, Alexander R., and Burhenne, H. Joachim (Eds.): *Alimentary Tract Roentgenology.* St. Louis, Mosby, 1967, 2 volumes.

Marshak, Richard H., and Lindner, Arthur E.: *Radiology of the Small Intestine.* Philadelphia, Saunders, 1970.

McCort, James J.: *Radiographic Examination of Blunt Abdominal Trauma.* Philadelphia, Saunders, 1966.

Singleton, Edward B.: *X-ray Diagnosis of the Alimentary Tract in Infants and Children.* Chicago, Year Book, 1959.

The Radiologic Clinics of North America, Vol. II, No. 1, April 1964.

THE FEMALE REPRODUCTIVE SYSTEM

Bishop, Paul A.: *Radiologic Studies of the Gravid Uterus.* New York, Harper & Row, 1965.

The Radiologic Clinics of North America, Vol. V, No. 1, April 1967.

The Radiologic Clinics of North America, Vol. XII, No. 1, April 1974.

INDEX

INDICATIONS AND ALTERNATIVES IN X-RAY DIAGNOSIS

This illustrated volume describes and depicts the various kinds of roentgenologic examinations available for the unravelling of diagnostic problems. The book is divided into chapters based upon organ systems, and the common abnormalities are illustrated. Emphasis is on providing the reader with a thorough background in the uses to which the ordinary and special x-ray studies may be put, with alternatives emphasized when the indicated examination cannot be performed or when more than one kind of examination is available for the solution of a specific problem. Indications and contra-indications are carefully defined.

This volume is ideal as a textbook for the core course in diagnostic roentgenology for medical students. Mastery of its contents should permit students beginning their intensive ward and clinic experience to select the appropriate diagnostic roentgenologic examination according to the indications presented by the patient. Moreover, a certain facility in film interpretation and differential diagnosis should come with a study of this text. The organ system chapters can be rapidly consulted for the kinds of examination available for study of symptom complexes of the patient.

The other large group of people for whom this work has been especially prepared is interns and residents in fields other than radiology. As a reference work to aid in the planning of a diagnostic workup this volume will be found especially handy, and its use may serve to reduce the number of non-indicated examinations ordered while pinpointing the patient's problem early in the diagnostic workup. While it is recognized that differences of opinion exist regarding the choice of examination in certain circumstances, use of this book should narrow the possibilities to a reasonable few and enable the house officer in internal medicine, surgery, pediatrics and obstetrics and gynecology to proceed with logic and dispatch in the solution of his patients' problems.

The family physician who is regularly confronted with the problem of deciphering his patients' complaints will find the suggestions in this volume useful in narrowing the needed examinations to those most likely to be productive of diagnostic information on the basis of which therapy may be undertaken. Its concise descriptions and explanations and its carefully selected illustrations provide a maximum of information in a minimum of space, allowing the busy practitioner to refer to the volume for guidance as frequently as necessary.

The material included in this book has been the basis for the teaching of medical students, house officers and general physicians for several years. It has been revised and updated frequently. This book is a modern guide to the effective employment of roentgenologic studies in the solution of diagnostic problems.

CHARLES C THOMAS • PUBLISHER • SPRINGFIELD • ILLINOIS